5 GEARS DIET

Learn how to drive your body

Diana Artene

Copyright © 2013 Diana Artene

First Edition: January 2013
ISBN: 978-973014115-3
ISBN (eBook): 978-973014110-8

Let your conscience be your guide!

Jiminy Cricket

Disclaimer:

This book is intended as a general reference only, and is not to be used as a substitute for medical advice or treatment. Nutritional needs vary from person to person depending on age, sex, physical activity level and general health status. The information contained in this book is not intended to prevent, diagnose, treat or cure any medical disorder. I urge you to consult your doctor regarding any individual medical conditions or specific health related issues or questions.

The resources listed in this guide are not intended to be fully systematic or complete, nor does inclusion here imply any recommendations or warranties, expressed or implied, about the individual utility of the information and resources contained herein. Your personal outcome will be entirely generated by your own actions.

CONTENTS

INTRODUCTION

Until 1980, less than one in ten people were obese. Worldwide obesity doubled since 1980.[1] Today:

1.5 billion people are overweight;

1 billion are dieters; and

0.5 billion are obese.[2]

"If nothing is done to reverse the epidemic, it is projected that more than 1 billion adults will be obese by 2030."[3]

The weight-loss industry was worth $385.1 billion in 2010 and is expected to be making a $650.9 billion profit by 2015.[4] Despite this huge increase in profits, there has been no sign of retrenchment in the obesity epidemic. The rates of chronic diseases, such as diabetes and high blood pressure, are also increasing in most countries across the globe.[5] The profit forecasts of the weight loss industry are based on the fact that people will become fatter and buy more weight loss products, not on the idea that people will become slimmer and not need their products anymore.[6] Fat people are paying their employees' salaries. So, their marketing departments work hard to make sure you'll need their products more and more each day.

-   And what are they really selling?

A dream.

Anyone can control and even lower their weight for a short period of time. You clench your teeth and eat only eggs and grapefruit, drink only lemonade, or take a bunch of pills to lose 5 pounds in a week. Amazing!

-   Right?

You can find dozens of free diets online, in fashion magazines, or in the local newspaper. And if, by chance, you live in an area without any media whatsoever, you can still ask anybody you might meet to recommend you a diet; be pretty sure they'll know of one. From hairstylists to dentists, everyone knows about diets. Everyone, unfortunately including many medical professionals,[7] will be able to recite one of the trendy diets they've heard or read about, perhaps one on which some famous celebrity lost weight. Maybe they will even tell you about their own turbid dieting past. Everyone is good at dieting, just as everyone is good at advising about how other people's children should be raised. Doctors paid by pharmaceutical companies to sell weight loss drugs, doctors and "nutritionists" engaged in weight loss MLM systems, and all the ready-to-help people in your life – everybody can tell you how to lose weight.

We are required to eat at certain times, regardless of hunger, and often told not to eat when we feel physically hungry. This social golden rule has brought humanity to the terrible paradox we live in today: half of us don't feed ourselves, because we cannot afford enough food; a quarter of us doesn't feed ourselves, because the food we eat is devoid of any real nutrients; the last quarter continuously oscillates between starvation and termite status. Thus, although there is an apparent abundance of food, today most people are dying of either starvation or overeating. For many people out there, food is their best friend, their greatest pleasure, and their greatest enemy. This completely chaotic "nutritional" world is an ever growing vortex, which will transform us into weight loss product slaves.

We live in a world of trends, completely accepted by an unconscious majority who do not realize that, even though the irresponsible embracing of other people's ideas might give them a warm life, it costs them their freedom of choice and their health. The freedom to eat what you want, when you are physically hungry, and to stop when you have had enough, is a right for which most people don't have enough motivation to fight. It is easier to follow the crowd.

As children, we are taught that if our knee hurts due to falling off a bicycle, a cake made by Grandma will make the pain go away. Indigestion passes as courtesy and is preferred by well-bred people. Literally. And so many well-intentioned people are willing to fuss over us with information about what, when, and how often we should eat, all with the fervor of a pilgrim in front of relics. I'd say that the "well-meaning" part is at most implied.

- Are these people interested in our short term well-being?
- Are they interested in the predictability of our eating patterns?
- Are they interested in our integration in the system?
- Are they "well-intentioned" toward our future health?

I am asking all these questions because there are a few simple truths these "experts" won't tell you. Simple truths that you might not even want to hear.

One such simple truth is that eating is not controlled by the conscious part of your brain.[8]

That is: you cannot control your digestive system, just like you cannot control your kidneys or lungs or heart. Just imagine if you could make your heart beat faster voluntarily. You could burn fat just lying around.

Another simple truth is that a lot of people eat when they are not hungry.

Hunger is a physical sensation that no one cares about. Many people don't even know it is a physical sensation. Moreover, a lot of overweight and obese people deny feeling physical hunger cues up to the point that they stop sensing it.[9] They eat because it is morning and it is healthy to eat breakfast. They eat because they are nice, polite guests. They eat because they feel happy and need to share, or they feel lonely, or sad, or angry.[10] They prefer to stick their heads in food, like ostriches in sand, every time they have a problem.

Some people eat just because they see a food that they are allowed to eat on the diet they follow. They are not responsible for the outcome of their eating: it was the doctor who said eating breakfast is healthy; it was the host who has spent all day cooking; or it was the neglectful boyfriend behind that diet fault.

-      These people have no guilt, right?

They are nice, or depressed, or happy, or just plain overweight and don't know how to handle it. They have a hard time expressing their love, so they share it by eating. They love to eat, but they are not thin enough, so they must hide their eating in order to not be judged. They have just eaten before the party, but they don't want to be considered disrespectful. They have a business lunch, so they must obey the protocol.

- Who cares about hunger?

Now, before you get angry and close this book without even reading the first chapter, let me ask you one simple question:

- To what extent would you control your need to urinate in any of the situations I've described above?
- See?

It's just a matter of priorities, ease and social protocol. I'm not going to tell you that it is easy to lose weight! Losing weight is simple, yet today it is the number one thing most people struggle with in life.[11] For now, please keep these words in your mind: priority, ease and social protocol.

This book is not about priorities. Not considering yourself as your own priority is simply unintelligent. Taking care of other people instead of taking care of yourself is doing what's easy instead of what's right. But, for many people out there, taking care of themselves feels odd. Well... no one will take better care of you than you currently do. If you treat yourself badly, so will everybody else. As a grownup, you must assume the responsibility of taking care of yourself, so that you have something to share with others besides frustration and anger. Offering to drive someone home with a broken car doesn't help anybody, because it puts everyone in danger.

This book is not about social protocol. Social protocol is a matter of power. There will always be times when you obey it, because you have to. If you have a hard time feeding yourself when you need to and not eating when there is no need to feed your body, then you'll have to find your own motivations to disobey social protocol.

This book is about making fat loss crystal clear.

CHAPTER 1: LOSING FAT IS SIMPLE, NOT EASY!

Let's imagine the fat loss process as driving a 5-geared manual transmission car. You start your car in the first gear, but you must shift to the second pretty fast; most of us just drive in the third or fourth gear. Of course, there are the more experienced drivers who usually drive in the fifth gear, and also there are the crazy ones who drive too fast and slalom without the appropriate driving skills causing the most car accidents. But for most people, the third and the fourth gears are enough. Now let's go back to real fat loss, long term weight management and beautiful, healthy bodies and minds.

Let me tell you how to use this book. The Gears do not provide "rules" for a full day, except for the Second Gear, which you must use once a day, every other day, in order to speed up a bit your fat burning engine. Every time you feel the need to eat, you'll have to decide in what Gear you'll "drive" during that meal. So, Gears are not "diet rules" for a day, but "fat loss guidelines" for independent meals. You can drive in the Fifth Gear when you feel hungry in the morning, slow down to the Fourth at a late business lunch and even stop your car completely for a dinner with your honey. It's up to you, exactly as it is when driving real cars.

And exactly as it is when driving real cars, the time you spend getting to your own destination depends on your commitment to improve your "driving" skills.

But start small: learn to start your engine and to use your brakes. This is essential, even when learning to drive real cars. And, because it isn't safe to actually drive your body faster before mastering these two skills, I consider of the greatest importance to practice the First Gear for at least 1 or 2 weeks before considering moving to any of the upper Gears. The info in this book isn't going to drive you anywhere unless applied. I can guide you to change, I can help you persevere through any possible relapses if you ask for my help, but I cannot change your body. You must do the work; only you can change it! So, perform each new small-step goal until it becomes a habit. So, only after mastering the First Gear, start to gradually speed up relying only on yourself.

You can shift back to a lower Gear if you need to give way to a loved one or to a hard working day. You can stop at a red-light event and restart your engine in the First Gear if you need to. Because the truth of the matter is that you cannot constantly be on one diet. No matter how trendy or easy or healthy a diet plan can be, it will not suit every day of your life, and it will not suit your mood shifts. You cannot eat only what is healthy and enough to survive. Sometimes, you'll need to stop. And sometimes you'll need and want to drive faster. This is how humans function.

As soon as you learn how to drive your body in the first two Gears, not only will you become a much happier person, but you'll also look and feel better. In addition, driving your body in these lower Gears will take the self-blame out of your eating. But first you must go through the learning and practicing phase.

Each upper Gear holds mandatory all rules of the lower Gears.

So, driving in the Third Gear means to apply every rule of the First and Second, plus the rules of the Third. Apply the rules, allow yourself the time to learn and get comfortable with each Gear, shift forward, shift back, stop, and restart. Take your time to really feel your body, hear its engine, and be in control. Then just keep going until you get the same feeling that you had when you realized you had become a good driver.

Your current weight is just a fact and you should feel no shame about it. You can change this fact today, or tomorrow, or whenever you're ready to commit the necessary effort to follow the guidelines that will drive you to your goals.

- Would you ever feel judgmental about parking your car and not driving it for a while?

Comparing a parked car with a "parked" body could actually be the point where the comparison breaks down, because you cannot just pour gasoline into a parked car with a full tank; you must drive your car to empty the tank before you can "feed" it some more. But for argument's sake, let's continue the comparison.

So, your body is now a parked car, weighing 20 pounds or more than you would like, and you want to drive to your slimmer, healthier body.

For practical reasons, I will describe each of the losing fat Gears in detail, so you can shift back to any Gear you need, any time you need to, and have complete control over your weight from now on.

- Remember learning how to drive?

I don't know about you, but at first, most of us had a really hard time starting the engine, driving too slowly or abruptly pressing the brakes and stopping the car on a hill, or in the middle of an intersection.

God, learning how to drive a car with manual transmission can be quite a pain in the... well, you get the picture. If you were born with a talent for driving, maybe you don't really get what I mean, so you should ask your sister, or your wife. Trust me, I'm a woman.

Learning how to drive is damn hard, and after you learn and after you get the driver's license, you find yourself alone with the engine stopped, again, in the middle of the intersection. But, every single time you drive, it gets easier, as you get better at it. And so it is with fat loss and weight management after fat loss.

So, let's get rolling!

Let's learn how to drive our bodies!

BEFORE YOU START YOUR ENGINE...

CHAPTER 2: DO YOU NEED A MAP TO LEARN HOW TO DRIVE?

This book is meant to make you think about all the lies you're buying about weight loss. I will ask you many questions and the answers are yours to keep. Just bear in mind that whether you answer them or not, you will still live with the consequences of your unconscious responses. So, here we go:

-   Do you need a map to learn how to drive?
-   Pretty stupid question, right?

But, in terms of fat loss, the "food guide" is like a map. It is important if you know how to drive and don't know the road, but still, it's just a map. A map doesn't teach you how to start your engine or how to shift gears. A map doesn't move you from A to B; it just shows you the way or the ways to get where you want to go. It might as well show you where you will arrive if you step outside the path you initially choose to drive on. But, you need to know how to drive and where you are situated on the map before you set off.

Sadly, the "food guides" nowadays are just like the maps from the 15th century: unreliable – most of them, anyhow. Scientists assume lots of things; contradict themselves, and the obesity epidemic reality follows.[12] There is the English food guide, the Mediterranean food guide, the French food guide, and the Asian one. And I'm not talking about cuisine. I'm talking about what would be considered a healthy food plan in each of these geographical areas.

Also, knowing where the starting point is can be just as important as knowing where you want to go. An objective medical evaluation is considered to be the best starting point for any food guide. But, then psychologists come and put behavioral problems into question. And you just love to eat with your husband, or you feel lonely, or sad, or happy. However, most food guides don't give any consideration to how you feel and why you eat.[13] They just assume that you eat because you are hungry.

I do not believe in a "general" food guide, because there is no such thing. Following a "general" government accepted food guide could just as well harm our emotional or physical health.[14] We are humans, not robots. Yet, for some, following the food guide is more important than the health benefits they're getting from it. That is how orthorexia (obsession with eating healthy food) came into this world. That is what the people obsessed with healthy eating are all about: the "food guide."

But, the food guides are meant for health maintenance and are not guidelines for the treatment of any health condition, including obesity.[15] These guidelines do not address the special needs of individuals. Finally, believe it or not, scientific evidence does not support any generalized nutritional approaches. So, let's go back to defining the starting point: medical evaluation plus psychological (self) evaluation. That should be the starting point of any fat loss road. After defining the starting point, you should define your own destination.

I will never suggest a meal plan for a week, for a day or just for one meal, to anyone. It creates external dependence, all-or-nothing thinking, and guilt.[16] Following someone else's precise guidelines on what or when to eat increases the chances of becoming fatter in the long term.[17, 18] Anyone who wants to lose fat for good must take the hard road and assume the effort of listening to their own bodies. All I will do is help you to regain control over your eating.

A food guide is a map. It can tell you where you are and show you the road to where you want to go. But the only way to drive on a food guide is with a toy car. Driving a real car on a real road and getting where you want to go is a completely different story.

CHAPTER 3: SERVICE

Just as it is a good, safe idea to check your car before you set out on a long hard road, so it is to check your physical well-being before setting out on any fat loss or sports program. I cannot stress enough the importance of checking your health status before you start driving to fat loss.

It's crucial that you check with your doctor before starting this fat loss program!

Do some blood analysis to check your blood sugar, and blood levels of calcium, iron, triglycerides, total cholesterol/HDL cholesterol and LDL/HDL cholesterol ratio. Also you can do a fasting insulin test to diagnose insulin resistance.

But, please keep in mind that I'm not telling you to ask your doctor for a diet plan to help you lose weight. Most doctors' medical training on nutrition is low.[19] Most doctors don't learn about weight loss in medical schools. They learn about weight loss from

MLM companies selling weight loss products or from pharmaceutical industry's marketing training workshops. They know how to sell you weight loss, not how to guide you to lose fat. Besides, what most doctors know about nutrition is related to patients suffering from different metabolic disorders, not to fat loss related nutrition.[20] So, when asked about weight loss, most doctors out there will just chant a diet from the internet or recommend the latest trendy one they've read about.

I'm not saying that no doctor knows about nutrition. While some abuse people's trust and recklessly prescribe diet plans or pills that are potentially dangerous, others continue their studies outside medical schools and specialize in the field of nutrition and dietetics - but these are few. And spending more on diet pills and less on healthy food isn't going to solve the obesity problem.[21]

In my view, doctors without extensive training in nutrition should not be allowed by law to prescribe diets or diet pills to patients, as they are not trained to deal with the factors that build an unhealthy lifestyle. Obesity is a very complex matter and doctors cannot cure lifestyle. Dieticians, nutritionists, fitness experts and psychologists – together – are the ones who can.[22]

The reason I'm sending you to the doctor is to check if you suffer from any disease that requires medical treatment. I'm not going to stand here and tell you that obesity isn't a disease. I'm not going to tell you that being overweight does not imply real health hazards. However, even metabolic syndrome X, in which all of the medical analyses written above are increased or at least abnormal, is treated best through healthy eating, sports and proper lifestyle.[23]

All I'm saying is go to your doctor, check your health status, and ask his opinion on your ability to follow a fat loss program that involves healthy eating and physical activities. Your doctor knows your medical history and is therefore able to finely pinpoint the limits of your health. Follow his medical guidelines and take medication if you must.

But remember: there is no medication in the world that can cure lifestyle. Obesity is a health risk that can lead to life threatening diseases. It is caused by an unhealthy lifestyle and it can only be effectively treated in the long-term through rebuilding a healthy lifestyle. Life threatening diseases are treated with medication. Maintaining an unhealthy lifestyle and taking medication for life threatening diseases before you suffer from such diseases is just plain wrong.

Asking a doctor for a diet is like asking a mechanic how to get to your destination. He can fix your car if it's broken and he might give you some general guidelines about how to get there... especially if he has driven that road himself. But he won't get you there, and any special car oils or expensive gasoline he might recommend can at most ensure a faster speed.

- But ask yourself, can you control "the car" at a faster speed?
- And will your engine work as well if you fuel it with something it hasn't been designed to work on?
- Think about it, ok?

So, that you don't end up using the crowded subway   for   the   rest   of   your   life.

CHAPTER 4: PSYCHOLOGICAL EXAMINATION

Most people want to be slimmer, regardless of whether they really need to be or not. Body image is our subjective idea of how we look. In the thinness-obsessed world we are living in, negative body image has become a serious problem for numerous women, men and even children.[24]

Dissatisfaction with one's body is a highly encouraged "quality" that is often praised as part of one's character.

We are taught to see the fox in the fable as not good enough, even stupid, when she says the grapes are too sour. Who cares that the anatomic structure of a fox's body is not built to climb the vine, she's not wise for acknowledging and accepting her body, she's stupid, not good enough, and she's got no willpower. Somehow, if she tries harder, she will get to the grapes. Then she can be praised.

Although it can cause low self-esteem, depression[25] and obesity,[26] the "never good enough, must do better" way of thinking is acknowledged and accepted by the general public as a sign of strong willpower. The human body is constantly changing, but still we are encouraged to identify ourselves with its shape and size. And if someone has a negative body image, centered on weight and body shape, the only path to a better, happier life is learning to accept and appreciate their body the way it is now.[27]

So, lose fat if you really need to, learn to eat natural foods (sugar and fat are natural, too!) when you are hungry and engage in fun, regular physical activity that you can share with your friends or children. Stop doing sports "to lose weight." Do them for the fun of it and because it is a healthy habit to have. Don't go on some weird diet, or even on a "healthy food diet." Don't ban any food[28] – you can eat any food, even if it's "unhealthy," but keep it as an occasional treat and share it with friends and loved ones; don't feel guilty for satisfying your appetite. Don't count calories, points or fat grams. Don't set rigid rules for yourself, like not eating dinner or skipping breakfast or avoiding carbs. Don't punish your body with purging or over exercising if you overeat at times.[29] Forgive yourself!

The opposite of overeating isn't dieting.[30] The opposite of overeating is smart eating and smart training. To lose fat for good you must work smarter, not harder. Thus, if your body is "parked" right now, just start practicing your healthy eating patterns as soon as you can. Usually, waiting until tomorrow's clean start will end up in today's huge binge.[31] Think of food in terms of taste and health, rather than as a source of calories, points or fat for your body.

Also, try to accept that loosing body fat isn't the answer to all the problems you may have in your life. If you need professional help to solve your emotional problems, don't be embarrassed to call for it. Repressing negative feelings can be extremely unhealthy. Learn to allow yourself to feel and express anger and other "negative" feelings that society or your family has encouraged you to repress.

And, emphasize your attractiveness by wearing clothes that fit your body and make you feel good. The clothes should be made to fit your body, not the other way around!

- So what if you don't look like the skinny model on the cover of *Vogue*?
- Are you sure that she really looks like that, at all?
- Are you sure she's happy and enjoying a fulfilling life?

The only purpose of her thinness is that it makes her an excellent hanger for designer clothes. Look at the hangers in your wardrobe!

- Are they sexy and gorgeous?

The old saying "don't do what the priest does, follow what he's preaching" has just been updated to, "don't look like a designer, look like a designer says you should look."

- So why the heck should you be as skinny as a designer's promoted fashion model?

If you want to be as skinny as a model for your Facebook profile picture, you can always use Photoshop.

Many designers aren't skinny or even fit.

- So why do they emphasize such skinny looking models?

They allow themselves the luxury of liking their bodies, because no one is considering their bodies. They are the Gods of fashion, they define the concept of "looking good," and they have the power. But one does not have to be a designer in order to have a positive body image. We can empower ourselves! It is just a question of self respect.

One of the most important causes of obesity is that weight loss plans are as highly promoted as thin fashion models, fast food and diets.[32]

Please close your eyes for a moment and imagine a world where there are no diets!

- Would you ever overeat again?
- If there were no diets to rely on, would anyone be so careless with what they eat?

In such a world, overeating (defined as eating when you are not hungry or eating past satiation) would directly cause obesity. Now open your eyes, and see that we are actually living in such a world.

Against most people's beliefs, dieting and overeating are two sides of the same coin.[33] Most people who diet live maddening lives. They make themselves chronically hungry, overeat in response to cravings and then, panicking about a possible weight gain, they over-exercise, vomit, purge or skip some meals. After overeating, most people swear to be "good," which leads to more dieting. More dieting leads to more cravings and the cycle repeats over and over again, swallowing them in a vortex from which it is almost impossible to escape.[34] Also, if you quickly lose some or a lot of weight by eating less than you need for the proper function of your internal organs, almost all the weight lost is dehydration,[35] and the direct consequence of dieting is a lowered metabolism.[36]

The starting point for fat loss is not dieting, but feeding your body only when and for as long as you feel biological hunger.[37]

Of course, there are healthier foods that you can eat, but there are no "fat loss foods." Considering any food off limits or trying to limit access to "treats" encourages the desire to overeat these very items. Restricting some types of foods only makes people more likely to overeat when they are not hungry.[38] The stricter the restriction, the stronger the desire becomes to eat the prohibited food. Thus, the behavior associated with dieting sets the stage for a future lifetime weight loss struggle.[39] Dieters use food to "self-medicate," to overcome painful feelings and distress. They eat because of stress, and then stress themselves out over eating.

And although most people, scientists included, might only be able to sketchily describe a "normal eating behavior," there is such a thing as "disordered eating behavior." Disordered eating is a term used to describe a wide range of eating behaviors that do not meet the criteria for any specific eating disorder (anorexia, bulimia, or compulsive overeating). Many of these disordered eating patterns are socially accepted as a normal part of life and even encouraged in our diet-obsessed world.[40] Disordered eating patterns cover everything from

- exercise bulimia: overtraining after overeating;
- purging disorders: recurrent purging to control body weight in-between episodes of overeating;
- orthorexia nervosa: a maniacal obsession with healthy eating;
- lipophobia: a worldwide "recommended" disordered eating behavior, based on the

avoidance of fat containing foods;

- night eating syndrome: daily starvation or underfeeding, followed by overeating at night, with a diet consisting mainly of comfort foods high in carbohydrates and adulterated fats;
- selective eating disorder: eating a highly limited range of foods, the avoidance being based on texture, aroma, food groups and even specific brands; to
- "wannarexia": a "hot trend" found in skinny teenage girls think it will make them popular to claim they have anorexia. The distinction is that anorexics are not satisfied with their weight, and wannarexics are extremely pleased with their weight, considering their ability to imitate the anorexics lifestyle a high personal quality.

The admission that some people have eating problems that do not fit into regularly distinguished categories of eating disorder would make it possible for a larger proportion of the population to break free of the weight loss obsession. We need food for survival, just like we need air, water and sunlight. Food enables us to grow, fight disease, repair damaged tissues, and develop and maintain a healthy body. Food is the fuel we provide for our bodies, so they can function for us.

To lose fat and keep it off long-term, you have to make peace with food. Thus, before starting this or any other diet plan, read the lines below and try to objectively assess your readiness to change, your goals, and your current level of commitment to achieving those goals!

The Process of Change has six stages, each with different "Characteristics" and important "Actions to take" that will help you progress towards successfully attaining the ultimate goal: a slim, fit & healthy body. Please bear in mind that I did not make up the stages in the Process of Change; they have been tested and proven to be essential for the successful building of healthy habits by scientists.[41]

Now, you've just started to read this book, so only read the characteristics of each of the natural stages of change and assess your current stage. When you've finished reading the book, reassess your position and start applying the "Actions to take" relevant to your particular stage.

Any time you ever feel like quitting, confront your problem directly by reassessing your stage of change and by focusing on the adequate "Actions to take" without being self-judgmental.

Understanding the stages of this process is of huge help in keeping you on the road to fat loss![42]

So, here they are:

Pre-contemplation

Characteristics:

- You see no problem with your current behavior and have no intention to change.
- Some people around you might perceive your behavior as unhealthy and advise or try to force you to consider making a change.

Actions to take:

- Inform yourself about the health risks of your current eating behavior.
- Inform yourself about the potential benefits of the change.
- Evaluate any potential motivation to change.
- If you ever relapse into the Precontemplation stage, focus all your efforts on finding motivation[43] – and restart fast!

Contemplation

Characteristics:

- You admit that the change may be needed.
- You weigh-up the pros and cons of changing or remaining as you are.

Actions to take:

- If you commit to making the change, set a date to start.
- Start driving in the First Gear when that day

comes.

Preparation

Characteristics:
- You take timid or bolder initial steps.
- You set some goals.

Actions to take:
- Set mastering the rules of each Gear as intermediary small-step goals.
- Keep a log of your eating, recording how hungry and how satiated you are before and after each meal.
- I suggest driving in the First Gear until you have made it through at least one full week in which no meal was eaten without hunger. Then, and only then, move forward towards the Second Gear. Do the same when it comes of increasing your fat loss speed from the Second to the Third Gear.
- Do not hurry to the Top Gears until you are perfectly comfortable with applying the rules of the first three.
- Starting to "drive" directly in the Fourth or in Fifth Gear, before taking the time and practice needed to master the lower Gears, will, more likely than not, make you fall back to Precontemplation or quit all together.

- Focus on your motivation to change.
- Evaluate any possible obstacles that might impede you in making the change and brainstorm ways to overcome them.
- Reward yourself (with something other than food) each time you successfully reach an intermediary goal.

Action

Characteristics:
- You follow the guidelines and are very committed to making the change happen.

Actions to take:
- Start driving in the Fourth and Fifth gears, and analyze what happens to you.
- Manage emotional reactions to change.
- Keep your motivation high.
- Brainstorm solutions for overcoming unforeseen obstacles.

Maintenance/ Relapse

Characteristics:
- You strive to integrate your new behavior in your daily life.
- Many people that strive too hard may completely fall off and relapse straight to Precontemplation!
- A relapse is not voluntarily choosing to eat a meal without respecting even the rules of the

First Gear. **A relapse is an uncontrolled eating episode that triggers negative feelings, such as regret or the need to purge or over-exercise.**

Actions to take:
- You must really learn how to brake and then quickly come back to the same Gear you were driving in before braking, in order to be able to persevere through relapses.
- That is why it is essential to take your time and master each Gear before increasing your fat loss speed!
- Take your time to learn to drive your body, and this is going to be the last fat loss battle you'll ever have to fight.

Moving on

Characteristics:
- The former behavior is gone.
- The new healthier behavior is routine.
- You can drive through holidays and special events with the ease an experienced driver would feel when driving from highways to crowded cities or off-road.

Actions to take:
- After a period of six months to a year of

driving mainly in the Fourth and Fifth Gears without relapses, move on to improve other areas of your life.

Because you are reading this book, I would say that you are at least in the Contemplation stage of the fat loss process.

- What do you think?
- What is your current level of commitment to lowering your body fat percentage?

Evaluate yourself and take the appropriate actions that will help you move forward toward your goals. And always remember: this is a road! For now, teleportation only works in Star Trek and in computer games. Therefore, we actually have to drive ourselves from our current stage towards the next. It will take time and it will take effort!

- Are you ready to change?

First Gear

Small-step goal no. 1: **Eat only when and for as long as you are physically hungry.**

That's all the First Gear is about. But remember that it is the most difficult part for a complete beginner. The sad thing is, as any driver can tell you, you cannot drive in First Gear and actually get to a destination. Imagine how long it would take you to get to work driving in first gear!

For now, you will just warm up your engine and start driving. Also, what almost any driver can tell you is that driving in the first gear consumes the largest amount of fuel. So, at the same time you must quickly shift to upper Gears, understanding and accepting that beginning to learn how to drive is actually harder than driving itself.

Many inexperienced obese fat losers give up here; they either park their car or try to speed up by overtraining or going through proteic or hypocaloric diets, thereby damaging all the mechanisms behind their engine... and then they park their car. Please be smarter than that and don't park or damage your car. You want to drive all the way to your slim, healthy body. Keep that in mind!

CHAPTER 5: START YOUR FAT LOSS ENGINE

If you have no time or willpower to do anything else for fat loss, but still want to lose fat, this is the main rule you need to follow:

Never eat when you are not hungry or continue to eat past satiation.[44]

No fixed lunch or dinner hours, no eating because the food is delicious, or was cooked by your mother-in-law, or because it's Easter, or you are at an expensive restaurant and the food cost a lot, or because you might never eat this type of food again. If you are not hungry and you want to lose fat, don't eat.

If you do not feel or recognize the hunger sensation, start your fat-loss engine by not eating anything until you feel it. It will take some practice to recognize it, but eating only when hungry is an absolute must for fat loss.

Hunger is a physical sensation we feel in the middle upper abdominal area, just beneath the ribs' medial junction. It is not a headache and it is not lunch time or the need to share food with your loved ones. It is a clear physical sensation with different values of intensity. And just like the urge to urinate, when you don't need to go to the bathroom on the first signal, you don't need to eat on the first signal either. So, develop the habit to pause, close your eyes, and see if you feel anything in the stomach area **before** you eat anything.

We need food in order to survive physically, mentally and socially. One may feel the social burden of not eating food when everybody around eats, not just from his own point of view, but also from others.[45] There are lots of unwritten social rules we all follow, like accepting the host's food as a sign of respect. No one cares if you're hungry or not, because the food is a social symbol that encapsulates too many customs and emotions. You must eat so that you won't be considered rude. My advice: be rude, be selfish, you name it – just don't eat unless you're hungry!

The primary purpose of eating is to fuel your body. The whole idea of eating is purely selfish, because you will live with the consequences of your eating. Thank God that good food exists and also good friends to share it with. Just don't mix these two up. It is amazing when you are hungry to have healthy, delicious food to eat with your friends. But not such a great idea to eat without being hungry just because you are with your friends and healthy, delicious food is available. Real healthy eating is pure selfishness.

Now, it is time for a bit of "underneath the hood" education. The unconscious part of our brain, the hypothalamus, is the control center of our inner world: the autonomic world. All centers controlling digestion, excretion, thermo genesis, breathing, pleasure and the endocrine system are located in the hypothalamus. It holds an actual "picture" of us, so if we change that picture too rapidly with crash diets, it will backfire by commanding:

1. lower muscle activity to decrease energy costs (decreased metabolism),
2. important fat storage, so you don't die of starvation,
3. and increased hunger, to make you start noticing that you are putting your health in danger.[46]

I will explain it all in detail later in this book. Just keep in mind that the hunger center and the satiety center in the hypothalamus together control the eating process.

- May I repeat that these signals are not from the conscious part of the brain, the hypothalamus being the **unconscious** part of the brain?

The conscious part of our brains is not designed to even consider the eating process, but to deal with the exterior world. A newborn baby knows exactly when to eat and when to stop eating, but most parents don't respect his feelings of hunger, because he cannot communicate his needs and because they "know better." So, you were taught to eat breakfast, lunch and dinner at fixed intervals of the day, 3 or 2 or 5 times per day depending on your parents' imposed eating schedule.[47]

Every single person knows when it will be better for others to eat. But most people have no idea when or why they should eat. Many people don't even know exactly how biological hunger feels. I do not think you should eat 3, or 5, or 7 times a day.

-       How would I know what your hypothalamus knows?

And your hypothalamus, as does mine, receives different stimuli from day to day according to each day's specific nutrient usage. The need for nutrients varies a lot from person to person, and even in the same person from day to day. Therefore, if someone wants to lose fat for good, the best, the hardest and the only thing that works in the long run is to eat only when and for as long as hunger is present. And then forget all about eating and about food, and focus on whatever they should be doing during their day. If you don't let your hypothalamus do its job you will diet again, and again, and again, without long-term success.[48] So, it is far more efficient and effective to simply stop interfering!

When you do feel the hunger sensation, try to eat as normally as you can. Do not wait another hour until lunch time, but also do not obsess about eating in the next 20 seconds. Just feed yourself as fast as you would feed your hungry child.

- Would you let your hungry child wait until morning and skip dinner to lose some weight?

Also, please try to eat at the table, sitting down and from a beautiful dish: one reserved for the most exquisite guest. And focus on savoring your food and try not to engage in any other activity besides eating.

- I mean, really, would you watch TV during Christmas dinner?

Don't spoil your eating pleasure by distracting your attention away from it!

Eat with the same awareness you would use while driving, to acknowledge when hunger stops.

Let's think a bit about snacking! The theory behind snacking is that these snacks will keep you from overeating at the next meal. But if you are not hungry, your blood sugar is not low enough for you to eat. Thus, when snacking, you start eating on a normal blood sugar. Even though you eat just a little bit of food, you can still raise your blood sugar higher than you would if you had low blood sugar before eating (equal hunger). The danger behind snacking is that you actually invite insulin into your blood without the pleasure, satiation and protective content of a full meal.[49] I will go into more detail about insulin in the next chapters.

Do not snack! Do not eat a piece of a cookie, some cheese or fruit just "because".

- Because what?
- Is there a law that states that you should snack?

If you are hungry, eat a full meal until hunger stops. If you are not hungry, don't eat. Allowing yourself to get hungry before eating is the first thing you can do to start losing fat and to protect yourself from regaining the lost fat.

The second thing you need to do to lose fat for good is to enjoy your food.[50] Always try to eat the tastiest and most satisfying food that you can possibly afford, when you are hungry. You can eat anything you want and if you really desire cake, eat it – but first wait until you feel hungry. It will taste better![51] Eating what you want, only when you are hungry feels like pampering your soul. Besides, the pleasure of eating will wipe away the frustration that usually comes along with fat loss and, with time, you will experience less cravings not more – as usually happens when you diet.

The last step of the fat loss equation is to stop when full. Some people eat beyond fullness, because they were educated not to throw away food. The only thing I have to say to people eating everything on their plates is:

- Are you garbage cans?

It is cheaper to walk away from the leftover food when you no longer feel hunger, than it is to literally and biologically pay for eating it.

Now, despite what most people think, if you actually give yourself permission to eat any food from the very beginning, it is easier to eat less of the food that you love.[52] But, you must give yourself permission to eat anything you like from the very start, before being hungry, before even considering fat loss. This intuitive way of eating is completely different than "giving in." Allowing yourself to eat what you want, when you're hungry is the foundation of your long term self control. With practice, as a very pleasant side effect, you will become satisfied with less food.

Never eat food that you don't like.

You might have the willpower to endure eating food that you dislike for the sake of weight loss, but many studies have repeatedly proven that fad diets have a lower adherence rate in the long run. And, as you might know by now, you will enjoy the benefits of any diet for a time, at most, equal with the time you were following that diet. So, if you do not want to start all over again every 2-3 months with the same or with a new diet, as so many people do, then just follow a diet that you can be on forever.

And never, ever go on a diet plan that you know from the very start you'll only be able to follow for a period of time, either longer or shorter. Continuously being on and off a diet is what makes food addictive, not food per se.[53] If you have any reason to think you will not be able to follow that diet as a part of your permanent lifestyle, then the best fat loss decision you can take is not to start it.

It's just like trying to climb a mountain with a heavy backpack. The heavier the rules of that diet, the heavier the backpack. Every time you fall off your diet, your backpack will roll downhill and you'll have to go down and get it. And then, you'll have to climb back up the mountain with an increasingly tired body and will. Repeat the cycle of the backpack falling off, descending to retrieve it and climbing back up again a few times and you'll just end up quitting altogether. You'll never want to hear about any peak. You'll be just fine in the valley, with no backpack to carry, if you know what I mean.

Now, I want to talk about another important fat

loss rule:

Don't plan meals in advance unless you really have to.

If you want cake, don't fool yourself into thinking that an apple would do. It won't! The only thing an apple would do when you want cake is harm. Trust your body! The more you trust it, the more in control of your eating you'll be.[54] The more you try to interfere with what you want to eat or with the hunger, the more you'll lose control over your eating. Thus, it is far more efficient to trust your body and escape from this weight loss obsessed world.

Let me ask you a question:

- Do you eat because of hunger?

Of course you do! If asked, most people say they eat because of hunger. But just keep a log for a week; write a "+" for every meal associated with hunger and a "–" for every time you eat without hunger. Then you'll see the truth! Only after such a week you can really know if your "fat burning engine" is on or off.

Also, before I teach you how to use the brakes of your car, let me warn you about self-fulfilling prophecies. If you are a chronic dieter who believes in miracle diets or a person who has counted calories since forever, then you will probably wait until you're hungry, because I said so and eat what you want, because I said so, but you won't stop when you're no longer hungry, because I haven't emphasized stopping enough. It is not going to be about you; it is going to be about me. It is not going to be about you losing fat; it is going to be about me being wrong.

I don't need you to prove me right and you don't need to prove me wrong. There is lots of science behind each concept presented in this book, thus don't bother trying to prove me wrong. This book is not about me being right. And, as I already said, if you have any reason to think that you cannot make this method part of your permanent lifestyle, it is best not to start it. That is because this method works to perfection if in any way you mean it to work. If you mean it to prove me wrong, and eat everything in sight just because you are "hungry," you will end up fatter than ever. But if you mean it to work, take your time and learn to listen to your own body by eating when you're hungry and stopping when you no longer feel hungry – then it will work.

Many women who have driving licenses think they are bad drivers, so they drive badly and then everybody just assumes that women are bad drivers. But there are also a few women out there who have really taken the time to learn how to drive and have practiced driving until it has become an important part of who they are. It is important because driving, just like being in control, makes you free. And it feels so good to be free!

CHAPTER 6: FUEL YOUR TANK

You are not what you eat, food is just fuel for your "car." You are the driver.

We need fuel for everything we do, conscious or unconscious. Even the body of a human in a coma consumes fuel in maintaining unconscious activities, like breathing or urinating. Your main reason for eating should be to fuel your body. But, you should stop eating when you feel that your body is signaling fullness, not when your conscious mind tells you that you have consumed enough calories. Doctors, dieticians, nutritionists and trainers could better spend their time highlighting the importance of hunger and satiation, rather than the importance of the caloric content of foods. Restriction of any macronutrient (protein, carbohydrate, or fat) is a potential health hazard and makes body weight maintenance after fat loss difficult. The more you concentrate on things other than hunger, the more you'll lose control.

Please remember that you can feel the hunger sensation in the middle of the upper abdominal area, beneath the lower medial front junction of the ribs; only after you feel something in that area you should look for food. In order to lose fat, always wait to feel physical hunger before eating.

Now, if you remember Pavlov's dog experiment,[55] then you must know that the digestive process starts when you see, smell or even think about food. The digestive juices are secreted long before the food gets to the small intestine, so they will be ready for use once food is inside the digestive tract.

- Will your body secrete the enzymes and hormones needed to digest sugar when you see, smell or even think of eating a "no sugar" artificially sweetened treat?

The sad answer is "Yes."[56] I will give you many sad answers in this book. It is up to you how you will use them.

Once inside the mouth, the food is chewed and moistened with saliva. The saliva contains ptyalin, an enzyme that starts the digestion of cooked starch by breaking it from polysaccharides into disaccharides. Then the masticated food passes through the esophagus into the stomach.

Contrary to popular belief, humans digest very

little in their stomachs. Inside the stomach, the hydrochloric acid and the gastric enzymes contained by the gastric juice start the digestion of proteins. There is a gastric lipase, but it is mostly important in newborns and not too efficient in adults.

So, sugar digestion starts in the mouth, whereas protein and emulsified fat digestion starts in the stomach. If we consider alcohol a sugar (and by the way, it is a sugar) then it is the only sugar that undergoes some sort of digestion in the stomach. Other sugars and un-emulsified fats are not digested in the stomach at all and even the digestion of proteins only **starts** here. What I need you to understand is that digestion mainly happens in the small intestine, not in the stomach.

And, as I will explain to you a bit later, if you separate eating carbohydrates, proteins and fats for the reason that they will remain "trapped" in the stomach if mixed together, you will get fatter than when eating complete meals, containing an assortment of carbs, fats, and proteins. The theory of separation is based on the "fact" that food is digested in the stomach. And food is not digested in the stomach, but in the small intestine.[57]

The stomach acts both as a warehouse and a blender. It blends the eaten food to small enough particles for the intestinal juices and bile enzymes to work on, stores these particles for variable amount of time, and then slowly releases only a bit at a time into the small intestine.

Emptying of the stomach starts about 30 minutes after a meal and is usually completed within 4 to 6 hours after eating. The result is gastric chyme, which is slowly pushed into the small intestine, only a little at a time and only when we're awake.

I will stop for a minute to explain why people that consider dinner as a "fattening" meal are both right and wrong. They are right in that it is not healthy to sleep immediately after dinner. But they are also wrong, in that it is not dinner per se that is unhealthy; it is not healthy to sleep after eating **any** meal.[58] Yes, you read that last sentence right: it is not a good idea to sleep after eating any meal, not only after eating dinner. Despite all the dieting "experts" who chant about how a calorie is a calorie, or about how we have better digestion during sleeping hours because we run on a parasympathetic nervous system, we can't benefit from a good sleep after eating.

In healthy individuals, the pyloric sphincter door between the stomach and the small intestine is mostly closed during sleep. And even when the pyloric sphincter is opened by the migrating motor complex waves during deep sleep, your body will still need to concentrate your blood flow on the internal organs, to remain alive. Keeping the blood focused on the digestive area during sleep, because of food presence in the gut, throws your internal hemodynamics into chaos and the last thing you'll have is a healthy sleep.[59]

People that go to sleep immediately after eating are usually people that, deliberately or not, don't allow themselves to eat when they feel physically hungry. They are so busy or focused on whatever they are doing that eating seems just a distraction. They usually associate eating with finishing strenuous mental or physical activities. Such busy people might look good or even fit on the outside, but many have high body fat percentage despite apparent slimness.[60] Going to sleep too soon after eating just provides a warm welcome to damaged gastric motility, irritable bowel syndrome and cardiovascular diseases.

To lose fat you must stay awake for 1 1/2 – 2 hours after eating, to allow the time needed for the blended food in the stomach to pass into the small intestine and start being digested.

Now, let me explain the "fattening" part of sleeping after eating. When you feel hungry for real, your blood sugar is low. Just eating and going straight to sleep is not enough to feed your cells. The food you've eaten just before sleeping will either be trapped in the stomach or will mostly be released from the stomach as bigger particles than can pass through the gut. Either way, most nutrients won't reach your hungry cells, as they need to be a certain size to pass through the gut wall.

And no, this is not the good news calorie counting dieters have been waiting for. Even though you might thank God that those "calories" haven't gotten to your cells, there are some cells in your body that cannot work on an energy deficit. The cells in your brain and internal organs need energy every second of their lives.

When you skip a meal or when you sleep after a meal, your body will take the much needed energy to feed your brain and internal organs from the liver cells' glycogen (glucose stores), **and seal your muscle cell membranes against glucose intake (insulin resistance)**.[61] Believe it or not, some scientists have even discovered that, because of the insulin resistance subsequent to starvation, you can develop diabetes through fasting or hypocaloric diets in which calorie intake is too low.[62]

Moreover, the next time you eat after skipping a meal, either by not eating or by sleeping after eating, you'll first replenish the glucose stores in your liver, and the cells of your brain and internal organs. Any leftover glucose will be transported to the adipose tissue, because your muscle cells have become insulin resistant, thus impermeable to glucose. I will explain this concept later in this book.

For now just know that when you sleep too

soon after eating, many of your "muscles' little soldiers" will be left without "food," so they will not fight for you. They will not die, but instead they will be unable to move. Each skeletal muscle cell deprived of glycogen just vegetates. It will no longer contract 24 hours in a row to maintain body tonus. It will no longer add to your metabolism. That is: skipping meals or sleeping after meals decreases your metabolism, making these fattening habits to have.

Sleep, healthy eating and physical activity are highly important for fat loss, but you must be sure to separate them in time to enjoy their benefits.

Sleep is very important for fat loss.

When you try to lose fat, but don't sleep enough, you don't just become too tired, cranky and eat more.[63] Deep within you, a hormonal army raised by your sleep deprivation will generate lipolysis and increase the circulating level of fatty acids, indirectly increasing muscle insulin resistance to spare the much needed glucose for the brain and internal organ use.[64] Therefore, you will decrease your metabolism and increase the levels of bad LDL cholesterol and triglycerides in your blood (dyslipidemia).[65, 66] You're not wasting your time when sleeping! You just keep your internal world at peace. Take my word for it: you do need your internal world at peace to lose fat.

So, sleep enough, but try to stay awake for at least 1-2 hours after eating, in order to allow your stomach to gently crumble the food into small enough particles and to start eliminating them into the small intestine.

There, the bile, the pancreatic juice and the intestinal juice perform the intestinal digestion. These enzymes can only work on small amounts of very finely blended food at a time. That is why in order for the nutrients to be properly digested and absorbed through the intestinal wall, the stomach must blend the food very well and it must be able to slowly release minute amounts of blended food (called gastric chyme) into the intestine. To cut a long intestinal digestion story short, the enzymes from these juices break down sugars, proteins and fatty acids into glucose, amino acids, glycerol and fatty acids able to pass through the intestinal wall. These nutrients are transported to the liver, to be processed and then released into the blood. Then, the blood carries oxygen and nutrients to cells, for use.

There is one more step before cells can actually use nutrients. Nutrients enter the cell's cytoplasm, but most can only be metabolized inside the mitochondria. This is a huge step that contradicts many diet theories. I will talk about this step later, in the Third Gear. For now, let's just assume that nutrients go straight to the mitochondrial system, even though this is not true at times.

The nutrients from the food we eat are not

transformed into calories, but into ATP (adenosine triphosphate), CO_2 and water. The mitochondrial systems of each cell transform glucose and fatty acids received through the blood into ATP energy. Calorie counting is futile and has nothing to do with real fat loss.[67] Please don't be offended and try to stay with me while I explain a bit about what "energy in" really means for the human body. A little science won't hurt you.

ATP is used in the cell as the main energy source for the majority of cellular functions. **ATP cannot be stored** – this is why eating more food to last longer between meals doesn't work for the body. Eating more food at one time will not supply the body with more energy, because the body cannot store ATP. The body can store nutrients, not energy! Storing fatty acids or glucose for future use does not equal storing energy, as nutrients must be transported through cellular membranes and then inside mitochondria to be eventually transformed into energy.

Having a nutrient stored somewhere in the body is useless if that nutrient cannot pass through the cellular membrane.

The idea of energy-in versus energy-out is only valid as long as muscle cells' membranes are permeable to glucose. And because eating past satiation increases blood sugar too much, the subsequent flood of excess nutrients and insulin will shut those membranes off to glucose.

To make matters worse, these membranes remain open for fatty acids, a fact that aggravates their insulin resistance further.[68]

Thus, when eating past satiation, the body transforms the excess food intake into fat and deposits it in the adipose cells. The crux of the issue is that all these mechanisms also happen when eating without hunger.

In English: focusing on staying within a "normal caloric intake", while eating regardless of physiological hunger, increases the body fat percentage and decreases metabolism even when the total body weight remains constant or when it decreases due to the dehydration associated with the metabolic decrease.[69]

We need glucose inside muscle cells to burn fatty acids up into ATP and lose weight. Taking fatty acids from the adipose cells and storing them inside muscle cells because glucose cannot pass through their membranes is not fat loss. It is water-weight loss, decreased metabolism, dyslipidemia, fatty liver, infertility, and many other ugly realities.[70] Eating when not hungry or past satiation cause obesity, not eating per se. So, eat when your body needs fueling, not before.

Now, going back to the energy, from oxidizing

one molecule of glucose, we theoretically get a maximum of 36 molecules of ATP. The majority of cellular ATP is generated by this process, glucose metabolism being the main process that human cells use to create energy. The other process is the metabolism of fatty acids.

Dozens of ATP molecules are generated by the complete metabolism of a single long-chain fatty acid. The high energy yield of this process might explain why human fat tissue is the densest store of energy. The problem is that this store is highly protected by the human body, which uses the best defense it's got to protect it: insulin. Fatty acids cannot be released from the adipose tissue as long as insulin is in the picture, because insulin inhibits the enzymes that perform lipolysis.[71]

Some think that they can lose fat by counting calories, by not eating carbohydrates, by skipping meals or by training longer. Chances are you will just increase your Michelin love handles, as long as you are feeding yourself regardless of hunger.

Moreover, every time you skip a meal associated with hunger, you will deplete muscle glucose stores (glycogen) while contracting skeletal muscles to maintain body tone, **and** block muscle glucose uptake – to redirect it to the cells of the brain and internal organs, which require it for survival. You will be left with a lower metabolism and with an increased appetite for whatever food is in sight and not tied down to the floor.[72] You will lose weight through dehydration.

But you will increase the fat percentage of your body. Each time you'll need to restart you'll need to go lower and lower on your daily caloric intake. You will become fatter than before, and fatter, and fatter with every too low calorie diet you attempt.

CHAPTER 7: HYPOCALORIC DIETS

Many scientists express food energy as calories. Also, in some civilized countries, it is mandatory by law to write the number of calories on the label of commercialized food products. Coincidentally, the levels of obesity in such countries are the highest in the world... and growing. Scientists think that putting numbers on the label of foods should help the population to lose weight. I think the opposite: calories are the scientists' way of dismissing fat people. It's like saying: "It's your fault, you fix it!"

But, being submissive and eating only the calories "allowed" by whatever diet you're following this season has nothing to do with fat loss. I consider calorie counting a totally ineffective fat loss hassle – potentially harmful in the long run – because of the food preoccupation it produces. And food preoccupation is the number one reason that people become diet slaves for life.[73]

Not eating when you really are hungry – because you have already finished your daily calorie budget or because you think that skipping meals will make you fit into your dream skinny jeans faster – can only make you fat on the inside. As I said in the previous chapter, if you don't feed yourself when you are physically hungry, your metabolic rate decreases. You become fatter "on the inside" despite the fact that on "the outside" your total body weight has decreased. And, in spite of the all prized Body Mass Index healthy range, many lean people with "healthy" BMI have high body fat percentage and subsequent high cardiovascular risk.[74] Thus, it is not enough to look lean, in order to be healthy you need to have a lower body fat percentage too.

The more you eat certain things at specified times, regardless of hunger, to decrease your "caloric intake," the higher your body fat percentage can become.

Also, you cannot eat both when hungry and when not hungry, without gaining fat. You have to somehow match the intake of food to the physical needs of your body – needs you won't know anything about unless you listen to it.

So, let's forget all about calories!

I hear your distrust.

I hear your fear.

But just use your brain!

The most recognized food energy unit, the (k)calorie, is not a human-specific unit of energy, it is just the amount of heat needed in the laboratory to raise the temperature of one kilogram of water by 1 °C. The caloric value of different foods is measured in the lab, not in the human body. You can actually measure the "caloric content" of a Christmas tree or of a shoebox.

These measurements do not take into account if you are starving yourself or if you have been underfeeding yourself for the past several months or if you are stressed.[75] They don't take into account that you might be ill, or even if it's summer or winter.[76] These measurements don't take your body, or any human body for that matter, into consideration. The conditions in the laboratory are standardized. Changing those standard conditions to mimic the human body's adaptation abilities would create even more chaos in the diet world. The human body does not have laboratory conditions. We are open physical systems. **We adapt.**

Therefore the energetic value that one particular food item can provide in a human body varies from body to body, it varies inside the same body from day to day,[77] and it can be completely different from the energetic value provided by the same food under standard laboratory conditions.[78]

- So what are you counting (for)?

- Do you think mathematics will solve your fat gain problem?

Even if the energy provided by a piece of food that contains X grams of fat, and Y grams of carbohydrates, and Z grams of proteins would be the same in the lab and hypothetically in all our bodies, let me tell you about another piece of this puzzle that doesn't fit.

Not all the nutrients from the food we eat are meant to be transformed into energy inside the human body.

I'm not going to speak about nutrients' bioavailability now. Just allow me to give you a crystal clear example so you can understand my point.

We almost never use protein as energy.

Yes, some amino acids can enter Krebs cycle (biochemical reactions that yield cellular energy) and generate ATP, but for sedentary people this only happens when cellular energy needs are met already, If cellular energy needs are not met, fatty acids (and not proteins) are delivered to cells for use – which is great – but we still need some carbs to "burn" those fats and get the energy.

Active people's muscle cells use proteins as energy when the inner muscular cells are left without carbohydrates. They burn fat as energy during low to moderate intensity aerobic exercises, carbohydrates during high intensity aerobic or anaerobic ones, and structural proteins after the carbs are finished. But this protein use for energy comes along with delayed onset muscle fever (that immense pain you feel in your muscles 2 to 4 days after performing exercises you're not accustomed with). So, if you want to know when to count proteins as caloric energy, simply wait for the pain.

Also, in the liver and in the kidney, glucagon (a pancreatic hormone that I will talk about a bit later) may transform some proteins into sugars through gluconeogenesis, so they can be used as energy when the going gets rough. But despite the fact that this process only happens when blood sugar is too low,[79] we are still "educated" to count the calories from the proteins as part of our "caloric intake." Whatever "caloric intake" might mean...

Here's another piece of this maddening puzzle that doesn't fit for humans. Human fat tissue contains about 87% pure fat. Following that 1g of fat should generate 9 calories, 1 kg of fat body tissue should equate to 7830 kcal. So, you should create a deficit or surplus of 7830 kcal between energy input and output in order to lose or gain 1 kg of body fat.

The reality is that if you eat 7830 kcal more than your body needs, you won't necessarily gain 1 kg of fat. You might gain more, you might gain less. A disciplined athlete might store those "calories" as glycogen in very active muscle cells.

- So, you see?

You cannot really know. No one can. My best bet is that you can never know when 7830 kcal will become "more" or that your perceived fat gain might be bigger than 1 kg if you are a chronic dieter[80].

- Can you really define what you'll look like if you gain 1 kg of fat?

In the same way, if you sum up a 7830 kcal caloric deficit during several hard days of eating less than the Basal Metabolic Rate (BMR), you might not lose 1kg of fat, since you might not bring into your body enough nutrients to feed the cells of your brain and internal organs, and so your body will go into starvation-generated insulin resistance, which will seal your fat stores. So, because of insulin resistance, even if you create an energy deficit of 7830 kcal, you might not lose one fat gram. Accordingly, in order to lose fat you have to avoid starvation and eat enough to at least feed your brain and internal organs. Any lower intake will shut off fat loss.

The complicated minds of the same scientists who associated calories with humans have taken one step forward in proving their intelligence when they brought to public attention the concept of Body Mass Index, which is pretty much irrelevant as a tool one can use to measure body fat percentage. About 25% of people with BMI within the "healthy" range have a high body fat percentage and increased cardiovascular risk.[81] Thus, the focus on lowering BMI can be useless, as it does not equal a decrease in either body fat percentage or cardiovascular risk.[82] On the other hand, doing a fasting insulin test to diagnose insulin resistance and focusing on treating or avoiding it, can make a world of a difference.

An old saying goes that "if you tell a lie a hundred times it will become the truth." Calorie and BMI "scientific recommendations" will make you fat one bite at a time. Buying any of these senseless "recommendations" should require a vow before God that would go: "I will never use my neurons until I get thin!" That is because using these "popular ideas" you can ensure that you will lose at least 1200-1400 grams of fat... from your brain.

Remaining on the funny side of science, let me tell you one more joke: After you lose some weight by following a hypocaloric diet, and you're satisfied with your hard earned new body, you will have a (s)lower metabolism. Thus, eating normal meals again, without the tiniest food excess, will slowly make you fatter than before.[83] And the joke's on you!

Remember: objects reflected in your car's mirrors are closer than they appear to be. And so is fat gain. Before the diet, you were fat, because you used to eat too much. After the hypocaloric diet you will become fatter by eating less.

-   So, how the heck can you lose fat then?

Exactly as you think you can: by consuming more energy than is provided by the food you eat. But the way to do this is not by counting calories; it is by **only** feeding your body when it asks for nutrients. Switch your focus on the inside of your body, to really feel what it needs.

Eating only when hungry stops fat gain, decreases cravings, cures food obsession, and prevents binge eating episodes. Then, regular physical activity starts fat loss and increases the chances of body weight maintenance after fat loss.[84]

I want to stop a bit to consider the thermic effect of food. If we really look into human body biophysics, we can see that human energetic output has two major components: the energy we use to stay alive and the energy we use to perform daily activities.

I do not consider the thermic effect of food to be different from the energy needed to stay alive. It is true that the energy needed by the body to digest food varies a little with the type of food that must be processed by our digestive system. But the energy used for digestion is a part of the energy expenditure used by internal organs and systems, each one with their own job. As kidney cells use energy for the excretion process, so the digestion system cells use energy for the digestion and absorption of foods.

However, the thermic effect of food was

presented by the scientific world as a big deal: imagine that even the digestive system's cells consume energy.

- Really?

This is incredible!

The logical effect of this breakthrough was the negative calorie foods theory.

- Would you eat a half a kilo of parsley or kiwi with every meal in order to lose weight?

These foods theoretically bring into the body less energy than is required for their digestion. Let's go with the flow and take kiwi as an example. After long, mind-blowing calculations, these "scientists" have established that a kiwi has a negative energetic balance of about 15 calories. This should mean that the body is using 15 more calories to digest a kiwi than the energy provided by the kiwi itself.

I'm not going to go into asking "whose" body they are talking about. Let's just consider that the human body functions like a standard lab and that the calorie theory does apply to humans. If we approximate 1 kg of kiwi to about 8 pieces of fruit, then you should eat about 65 kg of kiwi, in order to lose 1 kg of fat. Good appetite!

Most of the negative caloric foods are fruits and vegetables. Consuming them should be a health promoting habit, due to the antioxidants, fiber, vitamins, and minerals brought into the body. But any "too much of a good thing" is a bad thing.

So, yes, the fat loss process isn't instant. If you are a chronic dieter and if you've been messing with your body for some time now, you have to endure the time until it stops using insulin resistance to survive your diets. You might think that it's fighting you, but it's not. All your body is trying to do is remain alive. That is why next time you fail to take care of yourself and put your health in danger by going on another diet, it will take care of you by increasing your body fat percentage.

To understand more about why fat is so important for our survival; allow me to make a little analogy. Picture being low on money and you have two children: one eats just delicious, expensive foods and one would do with only bread and water, just to be with you.

- Which one would you send to the wealthy grandparents until you revive your financial life?

The human body's answer to this question is that it will send the pretentious child to the wealthy grandparents. This pretentious child is the muscle.

The body shuts of energy supplies to muscles when nutrient intake is scarce decreasing the energy needed to fit with what's available. It will try its best to never affect the energy needed by the brain and internal organs. It will put much of your skeletal muscle mass into insulin resistance to spare glucose for brain and internal organs to use.[85]

And it will simply not consider fat stores until it has to, because as insulin is in the picture, the enzymes that catalyze adipose fat burn are inactive.

The first place the body will cut down on expenses when famine arrives will always be the skeletal muscles, then the fat, then the internal organs and then you will die. But if the famine is not real, and it's just a temporary "weight loss" starvation, it will just decrease the number of active muscle cells in order to adapt to a lower energy intake.

Starvation equals a low metabolic rate, because it decreases the only variable in metabolism: the number of active skeletal muscle cells.

To better understand this mechanism, let's say, for instance, that you don't eat dinner, because you want to lose weight, although you are physically hungry. After you starve yourself, you'll remain with a lower number of active muscle cells to feed. Thus, the first time you eat after skipping that dinner will be perceived as overeating, because the nutrients will be able to enter into fewer muscle cells. And the subsequent energetic excess will go straight to your fat cells. Consequently, you haven't just decreased your number of active muscle cells, but you also have increased your fat stores. Now you will become fatter by eating less.

If you are fat, then you should find what drives you to eat past satiation, or what drives you to eat when you aren't hungry. You should put all your efforts into becoming aware of your eating patterns.

Other aspects of eating regardless of hunger are snacking and eating at fixed times during the day, so the body "trusts there is food around." Please, don't kid yourself! If you are not physiologically hungry, your body does not need any food intake. Therefore, hardly any food will be used to replenish the used nutrients, because nutrient usage was little in the first place. The Brain's, internal organs' and muscles' cells have a limited capacity to store nutrients. Thus, if you eat when their stores are full, the unrequested nutrients will be transformed into fat and deposited into the fat stores (obesity), into the muscle cells (insulin resistance), into the blood (dyslipidemia), and into the liver (steatosis). So, do yourself a favor: don't snack![86]

The truth is that low calorie diets create a nutrients deficit / muscle weight loss / slower metabolism / fat gain / **increased** caloric restriction dieting / even **slower** metabolism / **increased fat gain** vortex.[87]

If you live in such a vortex, please stop!

You are not in control of your weight, your hypothalamus is. And your hypothalamus is the – too busy to keep you alive – unconscious part of your brain. Counting calories with your conscious part of the brain makes zero difference on how the actual nutrients related to those calories will be used by your body.

CHAPTER 8: LEARN TO BRAKE

- What is the point of braking when you are driving to your best looking body ever?

My best bet is that you don't even want to think about braking.

- "Why lose the precious time?"

You've put your life on hold until you are thin and you don't want to waste one moment braking. I hear you. But take my word for it: learning how to lose fat for good requires the effort involved in learning how to brake first.

- "And what is braking anyway?"

Braking is simply allowing yourself to eat without hunger when you really need to.

- "WTF???"

Yes, I still hear you and I haven't lost my mind in the last five lines.

Besides allowing yourself to eat what you want when you are hungry, **you need to accept from the**

71

very beginning that there will be times when you'll need to brake, so you don't crash. Trust me, there will be times when you'll need and deliberately choose to eat without hunger.

I know the idea is hard to swallow. Encouraging you to eat when you're not hungry, after I have just said that eating only when hungry is a must for fat loss, seems crazy. But I'm not encouraging you to do anything. I'm not encouraging you to stop your car or to slow down your fat loss speed. I'm just saying that you must accept there will be times when you'll need to slow down and there will be times when you'll deliberately choose to stop for a while.

This is natural; this will happen for sure. Just as you slow down and drive with extra caution through intersections, as you slow down or stop when you give way or as you slow down when you drive on curves or on bumpy roads, so you will have to slow down or even stop your fat loss at times.

Please, think about it for a moment!

Being in a hurry or being a fast driver doesn't mean that you never use the brakes. Being a fast driver means that you control your car so well, that you are able to stop or slow down when you might need to avoid an obstacle **and rapidly shift back** to the same Gear you were driving in before.

If you really are in a hurry and you don't stop at the red light or give way to another car, you might get hit or even killed. So, braking is healthy and knowing how to smoothly brake is a part of driving fast. Just as you must be aware and careful when you slow down while driving a real car, so you must be when you eat without hunger.

- How much are you going to allow yourself to eat without hunger?

Only you can answer this question, and you'll have to answer it each time you need to stop or slow down.

- Do you want to park your car and not think about it until tomorrow, because you just had the worst day of your life and need a comforting dinner?

Go ahead!

You are free to do whatever you feel like doing. You will live with the consequences of your choice. You can choose not to stop at the red light, and you can choose to crash your car into a fir tree to celebrate Christmas. It's up to you.

The only thing I would advise you is to **only stop or slow down when you are happy,** because eating without hunger when you feel bad often triggers regret and binge eating.[88]

- I mean, if you're upset, frustrated or just plain low, isn't this enough?
- Do you really need to become fatter too?

When driving or eating, no one else but you is

responsible for your actions. Even if I were in your car as you were driving, you would still be in charge and I could do nothing.

You get to decide how much you eat when you're not hungry. You get to decide if you really need to eat without hunger. And you get to decide if there is no other thing which would best suit that particular moment that you can do besides eating.

You get to decide how long you'll drive slowly or how long your fat loss will be stopped. Just make sure you decide the moment you hit the brakes and hit them smoothly enough to have the time to make a decision.

For instance, if you've decided to stop the fat loss process by joining your girlfriends for cookies and coffee, be aware and carefully balance the pleasure with the consequences. Eat as many cookies as will satisfy you and as few as will cause the least harm to your fat loss process. Balance what you want and then decide. And trust me, this balance is easier to achieve when you're happy than when you're feeling low. What you need when feeling low is to take extra care of yourself, to eat healthily and to do some sport to pump up those happy endorphins into your brain. And always keep in mind that even when you "don't want to think about the consequences of your eating," you still have to live with them. Even ostriches do.

After you've braked or stopped, try to go on with your day as though nothing had ever happened and only eat again when you feel physically hungry. No guilt required. What you do require is awareness and the smoothness only practice can bring.[89] Therefore, if you need to slow down or stop the fat loss process, ask yourself if it's really important to you. You must ask yourself this question every single time, before stopping.

-   What is it about slowing down or stopping that serves you?

Asking this question is far less painful than asking "Why did I eat that?" So, stop being judgmental and start being on your own side at all times.

There are two days a year when we can do nothing: yesterday and tomorrow. All we have is now! And if now you need to slow down or stop, do it with awareness and get back on the fat loss track. Fast.

First Gear Recap:

Small-step goal no. 1: **Eat only when and only for as long as you are physically hungry.**
Never eat food that you dislike *
Sleep enough *

Although consciously braking is the basis of self-control, when it comes to building the habit of only eating when hungry, it is effective to consider it achieved only after a full week without any braking. Later on – when you have more "driving skills" and are better at controlling your "car" – brake whenever you feel it is necessary and quickly restart driving in the same Gear you were driving in before braking or stopping.

* These are not mandatory goals, but they might sabotage your fat loss unless taken into consideration.

Second Gear

Small-step goal no. 2: **Do 30 minutes of cardio/anaerobic exercises every other day.**

Get comfortable with the First Gear, shift to the Second Gear, and start practicing braking when you need to.

Don't hurry to get to the upper Gears!

Keep it safe and steady for as long as you need, until you feel confident enough to shift to a faster fat loss speed. Take your time and learn to be in control of your fat loss speed.

Also remember that this is not the time to go for leaner meats or to cut back on cookies. I know there is a little voice inside your head that just yells at you to eat diet foods to lose weight.

Don't listen!

It is just sabotaging you.

CHAPTER 9: HOW DID YOU GET FAT?

- What is the difference between a person who keeps their weight constant without effort and a person who has a tendency to gain weight despite repeated dieting?
- And how the heck did you get fatter just by smelling roses instead of eating of dinner?

Some say this huge difference is made by insulin and by the glycemic index or glycemic load of foods. They are both right and wrong. Let me explain why.

After eating, the glucose contained in the consumed food accumulates in the blood (postprandial hyperglycemia). Hyperglycemia endangers the functioning of the entire body if not controlled. Glycemic control is achieved through the secretion of pancreatic hormones, insulin and glucagon, according to the body's needs.

Ideally, blood glucose is transported into cells by

insulin, a process that leads to normalized blood sugar in about 2 hours, after eating only carbohydrates. However, the blood sugar levels are brought back down to their normal fasting level only when the prior eating level was low (this is what "hungry" really means for the body). If the blood sugar wasn't low enough to create hunger before eating, or if you ate past satiation, the after eating glycemic rise will be too high. Thus, the postprandial insulin secretion will be excessive.

If such eating behavior is repeated, the body adapts by generating an abnormal pattern of insulin response to meals, which is one of the earliest metabolic alterations that leads to obesity.[90]

Moreover, the excessive insulin secreted after unrequested meals leads to hypoglycemia. And the main ways we "feel" hypoglycemia are: intense sugar cravings and loss of self-control,[91] ravenous hunger, sweating, tremors, headaches and anxiety.[92] Thus, you will feel an initial increase in energy and mood as your blood sugar increases, sadly followed by fat storage, lethargy, more hunger and intense cravings. However, these symptoms are mostly not taken into consideration by people that have just eaten. Besides the abnormal excessive secretion of insulin after eating without first experiencing hunger, the fact that hypoglycemia has gained widespread acceptance is the second causal factor of obesity.[93]

Eating when not hungry and not eating when hungry set the stage for chronic dieting.

Once started, the snow-ball to obesity continues at the cellular level. You see, insulin is like a carrier that facilitates the entry of glucose into the muscle and adipose tissue. Of course, the cells of the liver, brain and other vital internal organs are fed with glucose, but they don't require insulin for glucose uptake through their membranes. Muscle and fat cells need insulin to carry glucose though their membranes.

However, when the blood sugar is too low, insulin cannot introduce glucose into skeletal muscle cells, as these cells must be kept impermeable to glucose, in order to spare it for the survival of the brain and of the internal organs[94].

Some say "not all obese people are insulin resistant," but insulin resistance is not a disease. It's a metabolic adaptive mechanism that ensures survival both during overeating and during starvation.[95] All humans use insulin resistance to survive for as long as danger is in the picture. When danger passes, you'll gradually get back to normal insulin secretion. Thus, to say that a person is or is not insulin resistant is just a matter of "now." Depending on that person's future eating behavior, this "label" can change.[96]

I want to stop a bit to explain why crash diets increase the body fat percentage. During starvation, adipose lipolysis (the first stage of fat burn) increases the amount of circulating fatty acids. But skeletal muscle cells overloaded with fatty acids become impermeable to glucose.[97] And because we need glucose inside the muscle cells to burn those fatty acids, the fat burn process stops. Other insulin signaling pathways, such as the one regulating protein metabolism, remain unaffected. This way, the body saves glucose for the use of the central nervous system and internal organs, while preventing structural proteins metabolization for energy, both of which are essential survival mechanisms. Accordingly, don't think that you "suffer" from insulin resistance, but that you actually "benefit" from insulin resistance.

It takes some time to decrease insulin resistance, but when you'll no longer need it, it will stop. And only when it will stop, you'll be able to lose fat for real.

Humans also develop insulin resistance when the dietary intake is too high or unsolicited by the body. But, insulin resistance happens after repeated excessive or unsolicited intake of any nutrient, not just after eating carbohydrates. Because of glucagon, insulin resistance happens even if you're on a low carb diet.[98] The high level of blood-circulating free fatty acids associated either with low fat, high carbohydrates diets or with ketogenic diets just increases the fat delivery to the liver and muscles, generating or aggravating insulin resistance. Therefore, in the case of repeated eating without hunger or repeated overeating (defined as eating past satiation), the insulin finds the muscle cells' doors closed. When that happens, insulin just takes all the leftover glucose to the adipose tissue, where glucose is used to synthesize glycerol.[99] The fatty acids delivered earlier from the liver and the newly formed glycerol, are transformed together into triglyceride within the adipocytes.[100] And like an upset and angry boss that just about had it for the day, insulin inhibits the breakdown of triglycerides in adipose tissue by inhibiting the intracellular lipases.[101]

Thus, as long as insulin resistance is in the picture, there can be no fat burning whatsoever.

When the glucose uptake was not requested by hunger or when you overeat no matter what, insulin will stimulate both accumulation of fat into your adipose tissue and will inhibit the release of fatty acids from the adipose tissue. And all this is done while your skeletal muscle cells are literally starving, despite overeating. You become fatter and fatter, while the number of your active muscle cells becomes smaller and smaller.

Every time you eat without being hungry, or you overeat, you follow this path and accumulate more fat, whilst also decreasing your metabolism.

Moreover, in time, even adipose cells may become insulin resistant.[102] This might happen because adipocytes become less sensitive to insulin as they accumulate more and more fat, or because the high fat accumulation messes with their mitochondria.[103] Either way, adipocytes do become insulin resistant after a while – leaving all the excess free fatty acids for the liver to use – thus generating dyslipidemia (increased LDL cholesterol and triglycerides blood levels)[104] and steatosis (accumulation of fatty acids in the liver).[105]

If eating when not hungry and not eating when hungry describes your way of life, you will become fatter and sicker no matter how many diets you follow or how many slimming pills you take. This is because your pancreas will secrete more insulin as a defense against your eating behavior, while your body will become more insulin resistant.

The larger new insulin army will try to forcibly introduce the glucose through the increasingly starving, closed muscle cell walls, and this will happen again and again, until you either run out of insulin and develop diabetes[106] or until you become so fat that you die.[107]

Although insulin resistance helps humans survive famine, with today's typical lifestyle of dieting, overeating and sedentarism, it leads to dyslipidemia, hypertension, obesity, diabetes, stroke, gout, polycystic ovary syndrome and subsequent infertility.

-    So, why are you doing this to yourself?

Every time you eat without hunger or continue to eat past satiation, you increase the amount of fat deposited into your adipose tissue, into your liver, onto your blood vessels and into your muscle cells; you decrease your metabolism by decreasing the muscles' ability to take up glucose. If you continue to eat regardless of hunger, bit by bit, you will become fatter, overweight, and then obese.

CHAPTER 10: HOW CAN YOU LOSE FAT?

- Does lipolysis mean fat loss?

Lipolysis actually means the breakdown of triglycerides, either dietary or from fat cells, into fatty acids and glycerol.[108] That's all.

Yes, it means that the fat stored in the adipose tissue is broken down, but this translates to body fat loss only if the muscle and adipose cells are not insulin resistant.[109] Furthermore, individuals with insulin resistant adipose cells have higher rates of lipolysis than their non-insulin resistant counterparts.

And even if the diet is right, and there is no insulin resistance in the picture, it doesn't mean fatty acids released through adipose lipolysis disappear into thin air. Lipolysis doesn't imply complete fatty acid usage by the body's cells. The sad truth is that lipolysis is either the first step of fat loss, or the aggravating stage of insulin resistance.

Breaking down adipose stored fat and storing fat in the blood (increased LDL cholesterol or triglycerides) or in the liver (steatosis) is highly unhealthy and is the causal factor of nonalcoholic fatty liver, cardiovascular disease and diabetes.[110]

The result of increased lipolysis is not fat loss, but an increase in circulating fatty acids.

Lipolysis does initiate fat loss, but as I've already explained in the last chapter, increased lipolysis and the subsequent increased circulating fatty acids shuts off the glucose uptake in the muscle cells.

- "So what?" some say. "Muscle cells will just burn fatty acids instead of glucose".

This is wishful thinking.

Muscle cells cannot burn fatty acids when their membranes are insulin resistant and thus impermeable to glucose.[111] Such insulin resistant muscle cells will burn structural proteins, not fats. Fat loss is equivalent to adipose stored fat being "burned" up to ATP (please read the First Gear again if you haven't understood by now what ATP is). A fatty acid "disappears" only when it has been completely transformed into ATP, CO_2 and water.[112]

Fat loss is a 3-step process: lipolysis, beta-oxidation, and Krebs cycle. In reality, the final step is the electron transport chain, but let's keep it simple. There is no need to know advanced biochemistry for you to understand how you can lose fat. Just carefully read this chapter. I know there will be some words that sound like "more science than you can handle," but try to understand the process behind those ugly words. I will try to make fat catabolism as short a story as possible. So, let's get started!

Through lipolysis, fat stored in adipocytes is broken down into fatty acids and glycerol by hormonally regulated lipases. Insulin can shut down fat loss by inhibiting this first stage. That is one of the reasons why it is so important to prevent or solve insulin resistance. But once insulin resistance has been decreased, humans still need fatty acids to go through beta-oxidation, and Krebs cycle to be able to lose fat, and we need them to take place **within the skeletal muscle cells** – because besides skeletal muscle cells, there are no other cells that can be influenced to increase the energy they use. Your brain cells, nephrons or other internal organs' cells cannot be influenced to use more fatty acids than they usually need.

The fatty acids released through lipolysis are transported to the body's cells for use. Introducing fatty acids of more than 12 carbons into the cell's cytoplasm is not enough for them to be burned. Such long chain fatty acids need transporters to get across the mitochondrial membrane.[113] They must be introduced by carnitine into the cells' mitochondria.

Yes, L-carnitine is important for fat loss.

But before you start popping up carnitine pills to lose fat, you must keep in mind that we can also get carnitine from meat, that scientific evidence behind carnitine supplements' efficacy for fat loss is low, that carnitine supplementation has water retain as a side effect, and that carnitine is really just a carrier.[114] Carnitine does introduce long chain fatty acids into the mitochondria, but here they still have to go through beta-oxidation and then through the Krebs cycle for you to lose fat.

Thus, **simply introducing fatty acids into a muscle cells is not enough to lose fat.** We need the fatty acids to enter cells' mitochondria and then to be completely metabolized through beta-oxidation and the Krebs cycle. And they mainly cannot be introduced into the Krebs cycle without an adequate inner cellular supply of a glucose metabolite called oxaloacetate. If the muscle cells don't have enough oxaloacetate, because the dietary intake of carbs was low enough or high enough to generate insulin resistance, then those fatty acids will simply be deposited within the muscle cell and increase its insulin resistance further.[115]

So, if the muscle cell is not insulin resistant and if the dietary glucose intake was at least enough to ensure a proper cellular supply of oxaloacetate, the fatty acids transported within the muscle cells' mitochondria enter the last stages of the fat loss.

Through beta-oxidation fatty acids are transformed into a very important metabolite called Acetyl-CoA. It is central to the metabolism of all nutrients, be they carbs, proteins or fats.

Please, stay with me! If you understand this chapter, you'll never buy any of the fish wives' stories that the weight loss industry is trying to sell to you. Also, it might be of huge help not to focus on the actual words, but on understanding the fat loss process. If it helps you, you might as well call Acetyl-Co-A "Mickey Mouse."

This Mickey Mouse cannot enter the last "room" where fat loss takes place if the muscle cell's glucose uptake wasn't enough to give him the key (oxaloacetate).[116] Without the key, more and more Mickey Mice huddle in the muscle cell leaving increasingly less space for "the key bearer"(glucose) to sneak into the cell.

During starvation or too low carb diets oxaloacetate is depleted, both because it is used by the liver and kidneys to make glucose (gluconeogenesis) and because the dietary glucose supply was too low to replace the used one.[117] Thus, starvation and too low carb diets stop fat loss by preventing fatty acids from entering the last step of the process.[118] Without oxaloacetate, they are transformed into ketone bodies.

That is why you must understand that the

presence of ketones equals stopped fat loss.[119]

Ketones can be transformed back to Acetyl-CoA, but Acetyl-CoA will always need oxaloacetate to enter the Krebs cycle and finish the fat loss process. Therefore, ketones are transported to the only cells that still have some oxaloacetate, being the foreground for glucose uptake: the cells of the brain and internal organs. These can adapt to use ketones,[120] but what this adaptation actually means is that their cells have a constant supply of oxaloacetate that can reintroduce ketones-derived-Acetyl-CoA back into the Krebs cycle.

Most organs can work just fine on ketones – except the liver, which does not have the enzyme needed to switch ketones back to Acetyl-CoA – as long as the intake of dietary proteins is enough to ensure gluconeogenesis (a glucagon regulated process through which glucose is made from some amino acids and glycerol). But, because of the muscles' insulin resistance, the newly formed glucose will always be delivered to the brain and internal organs, hence their inner cellular oxaloacetate supply will be enough to ensure survival during too low carb diets or famine.[121] However, muscle cells are insulin resistant during such times, so they don't get any glucose. They get fatty acids and ketones, but that only increases their insulin resistance and the subsequent ketosis further.

And, of course, as insulin is in the picture, the only source of ketones we can speak of is food. This line is true, because adipose cells lipolysis is inhibited by insulin, so these cells can only leak fatty acids in the presence of insulin when they've become insulin resistant themelves.[122] And this is very bad news for your cardiovascular system, for your liver and even for any children you give life to after your adipose tissue has become insulin resitant.[123]

You can successfully lose fat only if your carbohydrate intake is low enough not to generate insulin resistance and high enough to ensure the proper inner cellular supply of oxaloacetate.

So: too many carbs > too much insulin > fat loss doesn't start.

And: no carbs > no oxaloacetate > fat loss doesn't finish, aggravating insulin resistance.

Very low carb diets and starvation will always inhibit fat loss due to the subsequent insulin resistance and oxaloacetate shortage within skeletal muscle cells. Paradoxically, the metabolic decrease happens even when such diets are combined with vigorous exercise![124]

A lowered metabolism equals body fat gain and weight regain after the initial dehydration weight loss.

To sum up, the first factor that can stop fat loss is insulin resistance and the second is a carb intake that's too low. I'm not saying that you have to load up on cookies to lose fat. And I'm also not saying that low fat diets are fat loss diets. I'm saying that you have to eat enough carbs every day to **avoid** ketosis, and to be sure that the fatty acids – released through lipolysis and transformed into Acetyl-CoA through beta-oxidation – will enter the Krebs cycle, eventually being transformed into ATP, CO_2 and water.

Thus, to lose fat you must: avoid or solve insulin resistance by performing regular physical activity,[125] avoid excessive intake of any nutrient, and eat enough carbs to ensure a constant intracellular supply of oxaloacetate. This is the only biological method humans lose fat.

When you drive in the First Gear by eating only when and for as long as you feel hungry, you just keep all your body cells well fed, avoid insulin resistance and ketosis. You stop weight gain and start fat loss. But your "car" needs speed to get you anywhere.

Regular physical activity is a must for fat loss, both because it enhances muscle cell insulin sensitivity[126] and because it has the potential to increase the number of 24h active skeletal muscle cells, thus increasing metabolism.[127]

Not performing regular intense physical activity, or messing up any of the fat loss steps will just keep you fat.

CHAPTER 11: FUEL CONSUMPTION

Losing fat is all about building the right lifelong habits.[128] Therefore, I advise you to take it slow and learn to safely drive your body towards fat loss.

- How can obesity be treated?

This is a hard question with a surprisingly simple answer. It is something like the Columbus egg; the solution is the most obvious one. Eat only when you are hungry and take part in the physical activity that you enjoy most, not the one that "burns more calories." Of course, if you are a chess player, you should go out and run a little. Don't be afraid to really let go, because, left on its own, the body craves yoghurt, strawberries and tomatoes, not only fast food and cookies. A little faith in the body's wisdom is part of the "treatment."

As you might know, there are two main types of physical activity: fat burning cardio activities and muscle building anaerobic activities. I'd say ski, tennis, tae bo, pilates, yoga, step aerobics and bosu exercises are somewhere in between cardio and anaerobic activity, because these combine a cardio workout with bodyweight exercises like squats and lunges (effect highly increased if you add dumbbells to your cardio routine). So, if you play such sports regularly, then you will reap the benefits of both worlds.

The cardio activities, such as walking, running, jumping rope, baseball, soccer, aerobic classes, cycling, dancing, badminton or swimming are the activities that burn fat.[129]

The muscle cells use ATP for contractions. At the beginning of the workout, the ATP is produced by oxidizing the glucose from the muscle glycogen stores. When the glycogen stored within a muscle cell is used up (which tends to happen surprisingly fast!), we start to get ATP from fatty acid oxidation if that muscle cell has enough oxaloacetate and if that cells has enough oxygen (only glucose can be metabolized in anaerobic conditions, and we cannot make glucose out of fat). This process happens only during moderate intensity exercises. When you hit the anaerobic threshold you start burning carbs again (made at first from glycogen, then from lactic acid or from muscles' constituent proteins). I need you to understand that this is the only process that we can influence to burn fat and we can only influence it in active skeletal muscle cells.

If a muscle cell doesn't have enough oxaloacetate, it stops contracting and begins to deposit fatty acids within the mitochondria, becoming more insulin resistant. So again, in order to be able to lose fat, carbs must not be completely banned from the diet.

Word of caution: after sport, don't forget both not to eat before you get hungry and to eat as soon as you get hungry. I know they sound the same, but these are actually two different rules.

If you do not eat when you're hungry after cardio activities, because you think this is a smart way to lose weight, you might decrease your metabolism. That is because cardio activities don't trigger the same adaptive response that intense anaerobic activity does. Low intensity cardio doesn't require more muscle cells to be "called into work" by opening more blood capillaries to feed these new working muscle cells; only during more intensive exercise are these effects produced to adapt to the strength of the exercise. And cardio activities also don't prioritize the muscle cells that have empty glycogen stores for glycogen replenishment. In English: if reading books on a treadmill is your sport of choice, this might contribute to your fattening.

Low intensity, long, cardio exercises can at best make you fat & fit.[130] However, if you wish to be slim & fit, as well as to maintain these results in the long-term, you need to increase your metabolism, not the "calories" you use during a gym session.[131] So, I am totally against long, low intensity cardio activities!

If you want to increase sports' effectiveness, then by all means increase their intensity, not their duration.[132] Fun, intense cardio activities can burn fat, but long stale cardio activities will, at most, decrease your metabolism by decreasing the muscle cells glycogen stores and oxaloacetate supplies.

Interval training cardio is the best cardio there is,[133] but it is not suited for the Second Gear. I will introduce interval training in the Fifth Gear. For now, just choose a sport you know you will enjoy participating in long term and you'll become happier and thinner with each workout you properly perform.

In the beginning, low and moderate intensity cardio exercises facilitate lipolysis. However, as I have said, adipose lipolysis does not equal fat loss.[134] You may very well remain fat or become fatter if low intensity cardio is all you do to lose weight.

Moreover, please keep in mind that although taking part in sports can be perceived as a huge personal effort, physical activity cannot effectively generate fat loss on its own. Sports can increase metabolism, speed up the fat loss process and help you maintain your hard earned results **only if** the dietary intake is adequate to the body's needs. You cannot out-exercise a bad diet.

If you eat without hunger or past satiation no sports in the world will make you lose fat. Through sports alone, without the proper eating behavior, you will see very little result.[135] Thus, to avoid being disappointed by putting all your efforts into the sports part of the fat loss equation, it is imperative to take your time and master the First Gear before starting the Second one.

Anaerobic exercises (resistance training) like bodyweight exercises, fitness or bodybuilding, can increase metabolism and generate muscle cells hypertrophy.[136] Performing such exercises on a regular basis increases, maintains or replenishes the proper active muscle mass that will protect you against fattening.

-   Remember the "little muscle soldiers" that fight fat?

When the anaerobic exercises are intense and regular, and if you eat only when hungry,[137] you will start to replenish the glycogen stores and oxaloacetate supplies of more and more soldiers. Your muscle army will grow bigger and stronger, thus you'll increase your metabolism.

But losing fat only by performing anaerobic exercises, although possible, can take longer than most people would be willing to wait to see results. This happens mainly because fat metabolism requires oxygen, thus taking places only during the short time it takes for you to get over exercises with moderate resistance. When you get your anaerobic routine into the high resistance zone, fat burn stops and your muscle cells start working on carbohydrates (which are the only nutrients that can be burned without oxygen). Nevertheless, raising this anaerobic threshold through regular resistance training increases your sport performance and your metabolism.

Anaerobic exercises create an anabolic adaptive response from the body. Anabolic means you store nutrients in your cells, not that you burn them. Thus, what you achieve through anaerobic exercises is an increase in the number of active muscle cells. It is true that this increased number of cells will use more nutrients to maintain body tonus, but relying on tonus alone to lose fat is perceived as inefficient and disappointing by most people who wish to lose fat. Combining moderate to intense cardio exercise with anaerobic exercises creates a faster fat loss.[138]

Therefore, I strongly advise you to either alternate them, or regularly play the sports that combine them.

Some people think that sport increases the actual number of muscle cells. This is biologically impossible, unless a muscle has previously been injured.[139] Resistance training can only increase the number of **active muscle cells,** it does not affect their total number. Nevertheless, through training, we can increase the size of the ones we already have (muscle hypertrophy).[140]

The skeletal muscles in the body contract to maintain tonus. However, each skeletal muscle contracts only the minimum amount of cells required by the average effort that it is usually put to. Please allow me to make a little comparison to help you understand better the way in which we can increase the number of active skeletal muscle cells.

Let's say that a muscle has 100 cells (this is just a hypothetical example). If you usually use 20 cells to perform your regular daily tasks, then those 20 cells will be contracted 24 hours a day to maintain tonus. The blood vessels don't even open for the other 80 cells and their glycogen stores are not replenished, so they just "vegetate." The total metabolic rate in this case would be equal to the amount of energy constantly used by the brain and internal organs, plus the energy needed for these 20 muscle cells to maintain tonus.

If that same muscle is put to a task that requires a higher effort, it can either not perform the task, or it starts to tremor in order to perform the higher effort. The tremor is due to an unsynchronized contraction of the newly awakened muscle cells, so don't be embarrassed about it.[141]

During low to moderate intensity physical exercises, we use oxygen for energy-producing biochemical reactions, thus the name "aerobic." When the energy need is higher than the available oxygen supply, we continue to function through energy producing biochemical reactions that don't require oxygen, thus the name "anaerobic."

As I already said, the only nutrient which can be burned without oxygen is glucose. But anaerobic glycolysis has a very low effectiveness in producing ATP (~5% of the one of aerobic reactions). Besides producing little energy, anaerobic glycolysis produces lactic acid, which is transferred to the liver to be transformed into glucose, and then delivered back to the muscle for use (Cori cycle). Thus, the blood flow to muscles starts to increase and new capillaries open to make the slower flowing blood replenish **more muscle cells** with the newly formed glucose and with oxygen.[142]

But if the intensity of the exercise is too high, this mechanism does not keep up, and lactic acid builds up inside muscle cells. That is why after performing exercises that requires a high enough effort to start functioning in anaerobic mode, you might develop muscle fever, through which the body adapts temporarily to meet the requirements of the task.[143] And that is why muscle fever is a sign of increased metabolism.

If the higher effort is repeated, your body will eventually establish that it can no longer properly function with the initial 20 cells. So, it will constantly replenish the glycogen stores of 5 or 10 more muscle cells – if the sport is associated with adequate nutrition – feeding 25 or 30 little soldiers that will protect you against fat gain.

The only way you can increase or decrease your metabolism is by increasing or decreasing the number of skeletal muscle cells that contract 24 hours a day for body tonus.

Of course, if you become sedentary, your body might decide that 20 cells are too many for its needs, and it might reduce the number of full time tonic contracting muscle cells to 10 or 12.[144] Thus, an active person will always have a higher metabolism than a sedentary one.

Anaerobic activity is even more important with age, because we all are genetically programmed to lose active muscle mass as we grow old, through muscle mitochondria breakage. Regular anaerobic exercise is the only thing we can do to prevent the decrease in the number of active muscle cells associated with aging and to maintain a good metabolism over time.[145] Without anaerobic activity, maintaining a healthy weight over time, or even a proper bone structure, is nearly impossible.[146]

- So, do you want to lose fat for good?

Then, do your exercises regularly.

If the muscle activity is intense enough, your body will adapt, keeping more muscle cells well nourished and active throughout the whole day and night. This means you will use much more energy just by being alive.

Despite intensive marketing, no tea, pill or diet food will ever increase the number of active skeletal muscle cells, which is the only variable of the catabolic rate of your metabolism.[147] Such a miracle product does not exist.

Your daily intake of food must correlate with the physiological hunger, in order to avoid insulin resistance. Then, and only then, the human body will be allowed to use fat stores for energy, and it will do it only when, or more precisely **after** intense skeletal muscle activity is performed.[148]

Eating when and for as long as hunger is present does not increase metabolism, but it is a 'must', without which the body cannot even maintain a healthy metabolic rate. Every time you don't eat when you're hungry, because you have already eaten without being hungry, you decrease your metabolic rate.

So, feed yourself only when hungry and regularly perform anaerobic and moderate to intense cardio exercises – to lose fat and stay thin for good.

Now, I want to talk a bit about some of the weight loss industry's scams. Lately, some conmen within this industry made some naïve fat people believe that just through their heart beating faster, they might fit into one size smaller... Please, fill the blank spaces for me! A little question for thermogenic supplements users:

- Have you ever heard of ventricular tachyarrhythmia, variant angina, or ventricular fibrillation?[149]

Maintaining a constant body temperature is another thing they've tried to mess with. The theory is that you'll lose more weight by performing physical activities when you are cold or by drinking iced water during sports. It is true that the energy consumed to maintain a constant body temperature mainly comes from muscle contraction, but if you consider cold a catalyst for the effects of sport, please think again!

The perception-of-cold center is situated in the hypothalamus, near the hunger center. Thus, if you feel too cold, you will also feel hungrier.[150] If you regularly associate cold and sport, you will end up feeling hungry, because your cold center in the hypothalamus is overstimulated not because you ran out of nutrients. Chances are this sport and cold combination will just make you fatter by messing with your internal messages. Eating more than you actually need to because you feel cold might sound natural, but due to the subsequent insulin secretion, it blocks fat loss and stimulates fat gain.[151]

Besides assisting in fat loss, sport increases stamina[152] and the resistance to stress,[153] as well as decreasing anxiety.[154] Moreover, regular exercise is the most efficient way to lower bad cholesterol blood levels.[155] Thus, regular exercising can prevent cardiovascular diseases,[156] memory loss with age,[157] anovulatory infertility[158] or impotence.[159]

Many sedentary people develop abdominal obesity. The fat on the diaphragm muscle is pushing your heart higher than it's supposed to be and leaves it positioned at an incorrect angle. This means that the heart must work harder to push the blood into the blood vessels. Therefore you might develop a heart condition if you do not start to change your sedentary habits and do some regular sports to decrease the quantity of abdominal fat.[160] The best treatment for heart disease is prevention. So, to prevent heart disease focus on eating only when you are hungry and be as active as you can, whenever you can.

Body weight exercises are also excellent for preventing and treating osteoporosis.[161] Accompanied by walks or playing with grandchildren, body weight exercises are a fantastic way for elderly people to enjoy healthier bodies and minds.[162] And albeit some of overweight young people might think that the lines above do not apply to them, one day they will. Taking care of our bodies is a continuous job that we all must do until we die. Old or young, we must move to be healthy – literally.

If you cannot afford a gym pass or don't have the time for it on a weekly basis, maybe you can just make the effort to go just a few times. Ask a trainer to show you many abdominal exercises, push-ups, leg raises, squats or butt exercises and write them down, so as not to forget them. In addition, you can always check the internet for more inspiration, or play Sportacus with your children. However, keep in mind that a good trainer can keep you motivated, help you create a personalized workout plan, and teach you how to properly perform exercises and how to prevent injury.

About exercise timing, when first starting to develop the habit of exercising regularly, the time that you do it is not that significant. The important thing is to do those 30 minutes no matter what. You can even split them up into two or three shorter sessions, if this fits better into your week days, for example. But you have to do them!

And please choose different exercises from one day to another and focus on performing them as correctly as you possibly can.

There is no need to know or to count the theoretical caloric value you use up by doing sports activities. You'd just be wasting your time and this can even be perceived as a "license to splurge" after strenuous training sessions. It's better to concentrate on how you feel. If you feel ill or you hate the sport you are doing – stop! Physical activity is supposed to be fun, demanding, but healthy. You should feel strong, not ill.

However, to generate fat loss, both anaerobic exercises and cardio exercises must be done at the highest intensity at which you are able to perform during that particular workout.[163]

You have to do it like you mean it!

To maintain sports' efficacy, you will not need to do more than 30 minutes. Over time, just increasing the intensity of your workout will be enough.[164] Nevertheless, I'm not saying that you should not do more than these 30 minutes. Participating in a 50 minutes aerobics or resistance training class could be just fine, as most of these classes start and end with low intensity warm-up and cool-down exercises. However, performing high intensity sports for more than 60 minutes can be hard to do without risking injury or without decreasing the exercises' accuracy.

Also, as everyone knows, high intensity sports increase hunger. More hunger means more eating, possibly more muscle mass, but not necessarily less fat mass.[165] So, please take this into consideration before choosing to attend two consecutive sport classes.[166]

Another thing you need to consider is that eating soon after regular physical activity creates an anabolic response, which may not be in the best interest of people who are trying to lose fat rather than trying to build muscle mass.

This anabolic response is beneficial for people performing high intensity anaerobic exercises, during which both the intracellular glycogen stores of the muscle and the newly delivered glucose (made in the liver from the muscle's lactic acid) are not enough to perform the effort, thus the muscle cells start to feed on their constitutive proteins. But, eating after resistance training with the goal of muscle hypertrophy in mind is important only when exercising in the fasted state and only if you really worked out – if you know what I mean!

If your workout did not exceed a moderate level of effort, if it's routine for you, or it did not felt challenging then it's safer to forget about your post-workout snack. Also if you ate 1-2 hours before your resistance training, this is enough to prevent post-exercise muscle catabolism if you seek muscle growth. So, don't jump into the "anabolic window of opportunity," unless increased muscle mass is your goal, unless you worked out at a high intensity, and unless you haven't eaten for about 4-6 hours prior to the training session.[167]

Eating solid foods too soon after a workout can mess up your post-exercise hemodynamics, which is the movement of the blood to the body parts that require the most nutrients at that time. Humans literally focus blood in different parts of the body according to biological needs. For example, when we eat, we focus most of our blood to the small intestine absorption area for increased efficacy. Of course, the blood runs all over our bodies every given second, but we open more capillary blood vessels in those areas that the hypothalamus considers to have the greatest need. In those areas, and for limited periods of time, the blood flows more slowly. This is a normal, healthy mechanism that we all enjoy without thinking about it, and that pretty much ensures health.

So, when we eat we open more capillaries in the small intestine area. And during, and <u>after</u> we perform physical activity, we tend to open more capillaries in the muscle areas.[168] I have underlined the word "after," because what happens in our muscles after the exercise is even more important for fat loss than during the exercise itself.[169] We consume more calcium, oxygen and energy in relaxing a muscle than we use to contract it.[170]

Therefore, relaxing muscles after exercise requires blood to be focused in the muscle area. And eating requires blood to be focused in the digestive area. However, eating has a higher hemodynamic priority than muscle activity, so we always redirect the much needed blood from the muscle area to the digestive area when we eat. Consequently some of your after-exercise-glycogen-emptied-muscle-cells might remain empty because you have eaten solid foods too soon. So, don't do it unless you performed high intensity exercises on an empty stomach, 4-6 hours after a previous meal; if you ate something 1-2 hours before exercise, then wait to get hungry first. Then again, if you are an athlete or if you went way above your anaerobic threshold, drinking a sport drink or a carb & protein shake can take less time to absorb from your gut, minimizing the hemodynamic impact.

My point is: if you're not an athlete or a hard working trainer, you cannot afford to go on autopilot and blindly follow the "after a workout, eat as soon as you can" concept. If you did not exercised hard enough, it does not apply to you.

Fat loss is not mandatory, but a personal choice and it can only be achieved through understanding the processes behind it and by putting in the effort required to develop long-term habits. Taking care of yourself is a personal choice that you must make each day on the behalf of your body's health. We all know that criminals are taken to jail for harming or killing other people.

- Would your body sue you for sedentarism if it could?

CHAPTER 12: SLIMMING ELECTROTHERAPY

Lately, everywhere you look you can find spas or slimming centers offering myriads of slimming electrotherapy procedures. All you have to do is to endure the procedures and your butt will get smaller, your thighs will get firmer – just as your wallet shrinks. It's just like an (expensive) dream come true!

Some people might argue that slimming electrotherapy isn't that expensive, but as with every product, slimming electrotherapy is more or less expensive depending on the speed of the promised weight loss. I am writing about this subject in my book, because too many people out there hurl their hard earned money on such procedures. But I pretty much consider electrical slimming the same as hauling up your car.

- I mean, really, would you flaunt through town in a hauled up car?

First let me separate these procedures into two distinct sorts of 'therapy': slimming electrotherapy and slimming thermotherapy.

I will start with slimming thermotherapy. The basic concept behind slimming thermotherapy is either cold or heat body adaptation. As your common sense will tell you, and as I have already explained in the last chapter, an over stimulated cold perception center stimulates the hunger center in the hypothalamus. Endure cold slimming thermotherapy often enough and you'll just end up feeling like you could eat a cow.[171]

You might eliminate some toxins and even tremor a bit to create heat through muscle contractions, but this is pretty much it. Deep beneath your skin, your fat cells will be just fine. And let's assume that you're following a diet during the time you pay for such cold slimming "therapy." Your hunger will increase over time, both because of the diet and because of the cold thermotherapy procedure. Yet, you won't eat more, because you are on a diet. Therefore, your hormones will order lipolysis and you'll start breaking down adipocytes' fat, releasing fatty acids into your bloodstream. And yes, these fatty acids will be delivered to the liver and muscles for use. But although you are about to pop open a champagne bottle as you're reading these lines, you might want to wait a bit.

If you do not perform enough physical activity, **and** if you do not feed yourself when hungry, you will not have enough oxaloacetate within your muscle cells to burn those delivered fatty acids, thus you will accumulate them into your muscle cells, making these cells insulin resistant. Consequently your fat loss will stop and the levels of LDL cholesterol and triglycerides in your blood will increase; you might even start storing fatty acids in your liver.[172] Humans burn fatty acids during intense regular cardio exercise, not during trembling.

Everyone is so happy when they hear that they've managed to "get" to their fat stores or when they hear the "lipolysis" word.

As I've said, it's like a dream.

But if you do not perform regular cardio and anaerobic exercises, it will be an insulin resistance-fattening-dyslipidemia nightmare, for which you'll pay.

The next in line is warm, or should I say scorching, slimming thermotherapy. If you pay to endure such procedures, you are pretty much wasting your time, and your money, and, I should add, you are a bit masochistic.

I would sue you if I were your body!

But, I'm not your body. I'm me. And I must tell you that all you'll ever lose through heat slimming procedures will be water.[173]

- Will you shrink in size and fit into your "whatever you want to fit in"?

Yes.

- Will you lose fat?

No.

- Why would your body bother to enter lipolysis because it's hot?

Dehydration is fattening.

Yes, heat can over stimulate your heat perception nervous center, which in turn will stimulate your satiety center.[174] This can happen. But if your blood sugar becomes low and you don't eat, because your satiety center is overstimulated, you will not eat despite a real need for nutrients. Not eating due to heat related satiation might not sound or feel like skipping meals, but deep within your body, your brain and internal organs must have a constant supply of food.

- Guess what happens when that supply of food is endangered?

The muscle cell's insulin resistance pops up. Good-bye, fat loss!

I will explain to you in the Fourth Gear that dehydration is a huge reason for (over)eating. You might say: "There you go! I eat because of thirst." You might even drink a diet cola just to be sure your thirst is increased enough to stimulate the hunger in your hypothalamic center. However, playing ping-pong between your heat and thirst hypothalamic centers will just mess with your real perception of hunger. You will end up without a clue about when or why you're hungry. And this is the beginning of your dieting slavery.

- And for what?
- Is passivity so important to you that you are willing to endanger your health?
- Does it take less time or does it cost less money to pay for such procedures than to pay for a gym access?
- And if "it's easy" is your honest answer, are you so weak as to not be able to perform some physical exercises?

You are kidding no one but yourself.

About slimming electrotherapy: I would agree that there's a bit more science behind it than behind the slimming thermotherapy. But I am not here to praise the people that invented muscle electrostimulation or ultrasound therapy. They were brilliant! But they didn't mean it for weight loss. They meant it for physical rehabilitation, which is a completely different story. You are fat, not paralyzed. You can move your body. Electrifying your body to lose weight instead of going to the gym is like parking your car into a handicapped parking space.

One of the newest slimming electrotherapies is ultrasound cavitation. Ultrasounds are very powerful waves, which can be used as quite a useful tool for physical therapy. They are powerful enough to break adipose cells and to release the stored fat within them. This is true. But what you don't know, what the weight loss industry workers won't tell you, and what most scientist know is that any metabolic perturbation that leads to an increase of fatty acids within the muscle cells shuts them down and prevents their glucose intake. As I told you already, muscle cells filled with fatty acids become insulin resistant. So, don't pop open that champagne bottle unless you consider muscle insulin resistance and subsequent lowered metabolism, high cholesterol, high triglycerides blood levels, steatosis, cardiovascular disease, diabetes or even anovulatory infertility reasons enough to celebrate.

A cheaper, thus much more popular, electrotherapy procedure is muscle electrostimulation. Muscle electrostimulation is a passive form of contraction meant to help atrophic or paralyzed muscles. It acts pretty much like anaerobic exercises. It creates an adaptive anabolic response within the body. It is tonic to some extent.[175]

If 0 represents paralyzed muscle and a 5 represents a healthy muscle, you cannot really get beyond 2 only through muscle electrostimulation. A paralyzed person might tell you that a muscle with a 2 force cannot perform antigravity movements, thus muscle electrostimulation is really just an adjuvant in physical therapy, the real treatment being kinesiology (read: "physical exercises"). So, even paralyzed people must (be) move(d) to increase muscle force and tonus.

You might not have a clue what I'm talking about here, and you might not care. You see your muscles contracting during the electrostimulation procedure and you know this is in some way related to weight loss. If the calories theory were true, I would agree with you. But calories theory validity breaks when insulin resistance and nutrients bioavailability step into the picture.

In addition, the anabolic adaptive response you create during electrotherapy will make your body store, not burn, nutrients. So, if you do not alternate electrostimulation procedures with regular cardio exercises, you will not burn fat but store it into your muscles. And even if you do alternate electrostimulation procedures with regular cardio exercises, you would still have to not be on some starvation diet to be able to lose fat. You see, I'm always talking about fat loss, because weight loss is fattening if it's not fat loss.[176]

Yes, I know that's hard to understand.

But the only thing you need to understand is that in the <eating only when hungry + cardio +

anaerobic exercises> fat loss equation, at most you can replace anaerobic exercises with electro stimulation procedures. The rest of the fat loss equation stays the same. And if you modify the eating when hungry part by following some weird diet, or if you don't do your cardio, you will gain, not lose fat and possibly even while losing weight.[177]

I don't know about you, but for me, anaerobic exercises feel much more "right" than electrostimulation procedures.

- What do you think?

Second Gear Recap:

Small-step goal no. 1: **Eat only when and only for as long as you are biologically hungry.**

(This goal should be achieved and practiced on a daily basis for at least 1 week before starting to learn how to drive in the Second Gear).

Never eat food that you dislike *

Sleep enough *

Small-step goal no. 2: **Do 30 minutes of cardio/anaerobic exercises every other day.**

Don't use any thermo or electrical weight loss procedures *

* These are not mandatory goals, but they might sabotage your fat loss unless taken into consideration.

Third Gear

Small-step goal no. 3: **Eat both vegetal and animal food when hungry.**

Eating only an apple or only yoghurt is not enough for driving in the Third Gear. Every time you feel hungry, you should eat both animal and vegetal food to ensure you have an even blood sugar for a longer time after each meal. Don't focus on the quantity or on the percentage of these foods; just eat both when hungry and stop when you no longer feel hungry.

Driving mainly in the Third Gear can make you steadily lose about 5 pounds of fat per month, until you reach your healthy body fat percentage.

Please don't weigh yourself every single morning, it is bad for your morale. Rely on your clothes and on mirrors to tell you that you lost weight, not on the scales that also measure the weight of your bones, your muscles and your internal organs. You really should want to lose fat, not weight.

- What do you think your lover will do before making love to you: look at you or weigh you on the scales?

CHAPTER 13: LOW FAT DIETS

The belief that dietary fats make people fat is old. The belief that dietary fats make people develop high cholesterol is old and very well marketed by the low-fat food industry. The belief that eating low fat diets stimulates fat loss, as well as decreasing high LDL cholesterol associated health risks is old, unsupported either by reality or by scientific studies, and very well marketed by both the low-fat food industry and the pharmaceutical industry.[178] These are beliefs you are buying because they have been promoted to you every single day since you were born.[179]

Let's analyze the fat taboo!

Regarding fat health implications, we can classify fats into two big groups: nature-made fats and man-made fats. The nature-made saturated, monounsaturated and polyunsaturated fats are the healthy fats. The man-made fatty foods are the

121

unhealthy fatty acids: hydrogenated and partially hydrogenated plant oils of any kind, margarine and shortenings, refined oils (unless they say "virgin" or "cold pressed") and anything deep fried.

Trans-fats are industrially produced at extremely high pressures and temperatures, with added industrial solvents to promote the artificial hydrogenation. This makes the fat solid at room temperature and less likely to spoil. Thus, trans-fats increase the shelf life of commercial food products.[180] On the other hand, they pretty much decrease humans' "shelf life." Sadly they are used as a common ingredient in commercial baked goods (like crackers, biscuits, cookies and cakes), in fried foods (like donuts and chicken nuggets), in shortenings and commercial salad dressings and any type of margarine.[181]

Some say there is good margarine and bad margarine, but all margarines are less healthy than butter.[182] Even if the refined vegetable oils are not hydrogenated, they still undergo the high temperature, high pressure, solvent extraction, bleaching and deodorizing processes. Moreover, this refining process spoils most oils on the supermarket shelves. Soybean oil, corn oil, cottonseed oil, sunflower oil, canola, grape seeds and even adulterated olive oil have been damaged by this process.[183] The structure of the fats is damaged, the natural antioxidants destroyed, and many free radicals are created during this process.

Initially, trans fats (read: margarine and refined plant oils) were thought to be a healthy alternative to saturated fats (read: butter and animal fats), because they were unsaturated.[184] But in spite of the fact that today we know better, unbelievably, there are still some doctors thinking and recommending this "fact."

That was just a hypothesis, which has been proven wrong by the same pharmaceutical companies that tried to sell it to the world. When in the '90s the scientists were paid to test it, they made a startling discovery. Trans-fats both increase the bad LDL cholesterol and decrease the good HDL cholesterol.[185]

Low Density Lipoproteins are the "bad cholesterol", because they have the effect of sticking cholesterol to blood vessels, while High Density Lipoproteins are the "good cholesterol", because they carry LDL cholesterol back from the blood vessels to the liver for breakdown and excretion.

Many more studies over the years confirmed this and discovered even more: not only that the trans-fats increase the LDL and decrease HDL,[186] but they also increase triglycerides blood levels, causing inflammation.[187] The inflammation process, by which the body responds to injury, plays a key role in the formation of fatty blockages in blood vessels. A high triglyceride blood level contributes to the hardening of the arteries and thickening of the artery walls, which in turn increases the risk of stroke, heart attack and other cardiovascular diseases.[188]

The explosion of heart disease in the middle of the 20th century coincides with the increase in the use of hydrogenated fats and refined oils in the food supply. It took scientists about 40 years to put their hypothesis to test and another 15 years to recognize the results of the test. Nowadays, food manufacturers (but only in civilized countries) are required by the law to list trans-fats content on nutritional information labels. However, **amounts less than 0.5g per serving are listed as 0 grams of trans-fats on the food label.**[189]

- How many people eat only one serving?!

The natural fats are the ones that naturally occur in foods without any interference from man: the fats in olives, coconuts, seeds, avocados, walnuts, almonds, eggs, milk, fatty fish and meats. Fats from vegetal sources are mostly unsaturated and therefore liquid at room temperature, except for palm and coconut oil, which are excellent sources of saturated fats, very stable at high temperatures, and thus excellent for cooking[190]. Fats from animal sources contain a higher amount of saturated fat, and therefore are solid at room temperature.

The scientific world is full of doctors, nutritionists and fitness professionals who tell us it's a FACT that saturated fats are bad for us. This "fact" has actually never been scientifically proven. It's actually not a fact at all, but another hypothesis based on shallow clinical trials.

This idea goes all the way back to a flawed research from the 1950s where a guy named Ancel Keys published a paper that put the blame on saturated fat intake for the phenomena of increasing heart disease.[191] It was a flawed research, because to draw his conclusions he only used data from a limited sample of the population on whom data was available regarding fat consumption vs. heart disease death rate. Also he did not consider other factors, such as carbohydrate intake, stress or other lifestyle factors. His conclusions were a shot in the dark about the possible cause of heart disease. He had pointed a finger towards the only factor he had analyzed. Even so, his study has been cited ever since as definitive proof of the "fact" that saturated fats are bad for us.

- If these "experts" are right, and a low-saturated fat diet is the key to good health, then how come the Eskimo population and the Masai tribe in Africa, not to mention the Pacific Islanders or even Greek or French people, are even alive?

Traditional Pacific Islanders base their meals on

saturated coconut fat.[192] The Masai tribe in East Africa consumes only raw, full fat milk and meat.[193] The Eskimo population consumes up to ¾ of their total daily dietary intake from whale and seal saturated fat.[194] And the French are known both for their high fat gourmet food and for their low level of cardiovascular diseases.[195]

All these people on such high fat diets remain virtually free from heart disease, obesity and other modern degenerative diseases. That was, of course, until the Western diet with fast food, diet foods, fat-free milk products and lowering cholesterol drugs invaded their lives.

I do not promote high fat diets; extremes of any kind are harmful. But the truth is that – although saturated fat does increase the bad LDL cholesterol – it also increases the good HDL cholesterol, improving the overall cholesterol ratio.[196] Improving the LDL/HDL cholesterol ratio by increasing HDL is more important than just decreasing the LDL cholesterol.[197]

Besides, the total cholesterol is a useless number, the real problem being inflammation.[198] I would really go one step further and say that the HDL blood level is the main factor that matters when it comes to the cholesterol problem.[199] Of course, I also consider triglycerides and LDL cholesterol levels, but these are mostly influenced by carbohydrate intake, not by dietary fat intake.[200]

The most common types of saturated fat are: stearic, palmitic and lauric acid.

Research proves that stearic acid, found in cocoa and animal fat, has no negative impact on cardiovascular disease risks.[201, 202] The liver de-saturates stearic acid into oleic acid, an omega-9 fatty acid. Although beneficial for humans, omega-9 fatty acids are not considered essential fatty acids, because the omega-9 can be created by the human body. Oleic acid is the same monounsaturated fat which is found in the most "extra virgin" of olive oils.[203] Cocoa butter is a healthy natural fat, composed of approximately 59% saturated fat, mostly healthy stearic acid. Besides the natural antioxidants contained in cocoa, that is why dark chocolate consumption is beneficial to our health.[204]

Lacking in most diets, the saturated lauric acid found in coconut oil and human breast milk, increases HDL cholesterol level significantly, and it is more easily used for immediate energy instead of being stored as body fat.[205] Coconut oil is also excellent as cooking oil, because saturated fats are much more stable and do not oxidize easily like other polyunsaturated plants oils when exposed to heat and light.[206]

Actually, many studies sponsored by big drug companies failed to even prove that lowered LDL cholesterol levels ever translated into measurable medical health benefits.

I am at least skeptical about the bad effects on health of the intake of natural saturated fat sources and I'll always choose natural, full fat milk products and whole butter over any type of margarine or over low fat milk products. Because "low fat" means that the natural product has been damaged and the implied health benefits are long gone.[207]

- If all of these researchers have tried so hard over the years to point the finger at saturated fats, but have continued to fail to do so, what are the REAL culprits for heart diseases?

The real causes of heart diseases are:

1. hydrogenated plant oils;
2. animal meat coming from animals forcibly fattened up with antibiotics & hormones, fed with grains and not with grass (which causes inflammation inside the body and throws the omega6/omega3 balance out of whack);[208]
3. refined carbohydrates and trans fats contained in cookies, cakes, crackers, and in processed foods;[209]
4. smoking;[210]
5. stress;[211]
6. sedentarism;[212]
7. and obesity.[213]

Both excessive carbohydrate intake and excessive protein intake play a role in increasing blood glucose, blood fatty acids and insulin concentrations, independently or together. I am pointing this out because natural dietary saturated fats are usually replaced with an increase in carbohydrate content, either in manmade low fat foods or in low fat diets. Replacing natural foods high in saturated fat with low fat processed foods is far from healthy.

Eating low fat processed foods generates insulin mediated suppression of adipocytes lipolysis and insulin resistance,[214] first in the skeletal muscles and, in time, also in the adipose tissue. Some studies have even suggested that when the muscle mitochondrial system starts to be affected by the increased fatty acids' intracellular uptake, this is written into your genes, which you can pass on to your children.[215]

- So, now do you see the bigger picture?

It is not only about you. And it is not only about now. From where I stand, it is healthier to eat natural foods, be they naturally high or low in saturated fat, than to eat any processed food.

For example if we compare eating low fat dairies with whole fat dairies, the low fat ones increase blood sugar more steeply and lead to an increased glucose uptake by the liver. Here, insulin stimulates de novo lipogenesis, transforming glucose to fatty acids. Some of these new fatty acids will be transported to the adipose tissue, but others will be deposited in the liver and, in time, can generate steatosis (nonalcoholic fatty liver disease) or steatohepatitis.[216] Besides being deposited in the liver, other glucose-derived fatty acids will circulate throughout the body as triglycerides, causing the inflammation of blood vessels, and increasing the coronary heart disease risk.[217] Any leftover fatty acids will be deposited into skeletal muscle cells, causing them to become insulin resistant. Because of their higher carbohydrate content, low fat foods have the potential to stop fat loss and to cause fat gain.[218] Thus, next time you see a 0.1% milk or a "non-fat" ice cream, just back off and walk in the opposite direction.

Consuming natural full-fat milk products increases HDL cholesterol. In addition, whether full-fat dairies increase LDL cholesterol or not is a very controversial hypothesis, contradicted by a large body of unbiased scientific evidence from which I have already cited some studies above.

However, it is proven that the regular consumption of low fat foods can decrease HDL cholesterol, and increases both triglycerides and LDL cholesterol blood level potentially generating insulin resistance, obesity, diabetes, cardiovascular diseases and infertility.[219]

Take your pick!

I cannot think of anyone who would benefit

from such misconceptions beside the multi-billion dollar diet industry, low-fat foods industry and cholesterol-lowering pharmaceutical companies.[220] They might have been smashed out by their own studies, studies meant to prove them right, but the doctors were too busy to use those studies for the benefits of their patients. As I said before, if you tell a lie a thousand times, it becomes true.

The true FACT is that nature-made saturated fat is a neutral substance in the body and even beneficial at times, not a deadly risk factor for heart disease.

The only thing we should worry about is the healthiness of the animals that provided that meat, milk or other derived food products, the real problem being their content of hormones and antibiotics, not the saturated fat per se. If the saturated fat comes from a healthy, free range animal, then it is healthy for humans too. If it does not, it is not.

But there is no doubt about the benefits of unsaturated fat intake. Eating unsaturated fats is one of the best things we can do for our life quality, besides not smoking, exercising and resting regularly.

Unsaturated fat can be found mostly in extra virgin olive oil, raw nuts and raw seeds of any kind, wild fatty fish and seafood, algae, leafy greens and krill. Whole food sources are always the best, as processing and heating damage unsaturated fats.

Omega-3 and omega-6 are essential fatty acids, so named because the human body absolutely needs them, but it cannot manufacture them – thus we need to get them from our diet. When an essential nutrient is not brought into the body, the body cannot perform the biological functions associated with that nutrient and slowly becomes sick.

I want to linger a bit on the fact that both omega-3 and omega-6 are promoted together under the term "PUFA" or Poly Unsaturated Fatty Acids. Both omega-3 and omega-6 are families of unsaturated fatty acids, naming different monounsaturated and polyunsaturated fatty acids.

Omega-3 fatty acids are mainly monounsaturated, while omega-6 ones are mainly polyunsaturated. Promoting them together under the same "PUFA" term can be misleading and potentially harmful (I will explain why in a bit).

For now just know that although omega-3 fatty acids family does contain some polyunsaturated fatty acids, I will refer to them as "monounsaturated fatty acids," because the monounsaturated ones are the most abundant ones. Only the monounsaturated Omega-3 fatty acids lower the LDL cholesterol[221] and the triglyceride level;[222] increase HDL cholesterol;[223] enhance memory and overall cognitive performance;[224] reduce inflammation;[225] and appear to reduce free radical damage associated with some cancers and rheumatoid arthritis.[226]

On the other hand, the polyunsaturated fatty acids have different effects on the body than the monounsaturated fatty acids. And because Omega-6 family is mainly made out of polyunsaturated fatty acids, I will refer to them as "polyunsaturated fats" although they do contain a small amount of monounsaturated fats also. Although they are essential to the body being the precursors of prostaglandins, the polyunsaturated Omega-6 fatty acids decrease both LDL and HDL cholesterol levels, and they have proinflammatory and prothrombotic (blood clots formation) effects.[227] Thus, an excessive Omega-6 intake increases the risk of suffering from cardiovascular diseases, as inflammation and blood clotting are the main culprits behind these diseases, not the total cholesterol.[228]

While omega-3 and omega-6 perform complex actions within the body, what I need you to understand and always remember is that **omega-6 fatty acids lower the good HDL cholesterol, and that they have inflammatory and prothrombotic activity.** So, it is important to stop putting Omega-3 and Omega-6 under the same "PUFA" umbrella.

Thousands of years ago, the human diet consisted of approximately equal parts omega−3 and omega−6 essential fatty acids.[229] But, since the beginning of agriculture, there has been a steady increase in omega−6 at the expense of omega−3 fat in the diet. This process accelerated when animals began to be fed increasingly on grains, rather than grass. Furthermore, recommendations to eat plant fats rather than animal fats, or to replace butter with margarine or plant shortenings, increased the trend towards omega−6 and trans-fats consumption. At present, the ratio of omega−6 to omega−3 fatty acids in the western diet is 20:1 or more, the optimum ratio being below 4:1.[230]

This imbalanced omega-6 / omega-3 fatty acid ratio has led to increased prevalence of breast cancer,[231] cardiovascular diseases,[232] obesity,[233] diabetes,[234] and even of ADHD (attention deficit disorder) in children.[235]

The polyunsaturated omega-6 fatty acids come from foods like refined soybean oil and derived soy products; breakfast cereals; refined corn, rapeseed, canola or sunflower oils; and from grain-fed poultry meat and eggs, or cattle meat and dairy products coming from animals that were not allowed to feed naturally on grass, but forcibly fattened up with cereals. A diet based on polyunsaturated omega-6 fatty acids increases inflammation of blood vessels, increases blood clotting and decreases both HDL and LDL cholesterol levels. Thus, lowering the daily intake of omega-6 fatty acids is mandatory for our health and for the proper development of our children's bodies and minds.

Nevertheless, remember that omega-6 is a family of fatty acids essential for our health, which our body cannot create by itself. Thus you should not completely avoid it. As with everything, moderation is the key factor with the omega-6 intake.

Getting more monounsaturated omega-3 fatty acids from our diet helps us reduce inflammation and improve the risk of suffering from many subsequent diseases, such as colon cancer,[236] asthma,[237] or psychiatric disorders.[238] It also helps us regulate blood clotting[239] and keep the LDL/HDL cholesterol ratio at a healthy level, thus decreasing the risk of cardiovascular disease.[240]

Let me summarize this:

Trans-fats from margarines, commercial fried foods and cookies that contain hydrogenated fats (please read food labels!) increase LDL, decrease HDL and cause inflammation.

Polyunsaturated omega-6 fatty acids from most plant oils presented above, from soy, breakfast cereals and grain-fed poultry and cattle, decrease LDL, decrease HDL, and cause inflammation.

Saturated fats from grass-fed animals increase LDL, increase HDL, and have no proinflammatory properties.

Monounsaturated omega-3 fatty acids decrease LDL and increase HDL and reduce inflammation.

Extra virgin cold pressed olive oil (which comes from the first pressing of the olives), avocados, fatty fish (such as wild salmon, sardines, herring and trout), <u>raw</u> nuts, walnuts, and almonds are some of the many sources of monounsaturated omega-3 fats. Along with regular physical activity, eating such foods on a daily basis will increase your good HDL cholesterol and decrease your bad LDL cholesterol, helping you prevent cardiovascular diseases.

Avocado has the highest beneficial omega-3 fatty acid content of any fruit. But you have to eat it soon after cutting it, because omega-3 fats are highly reactive to light. For the same reason, freshly ground flax seed is the only way to consume them for an optimal omega-3 intake. In addition, because omega-3 fatty acids are also damaged by heat,[241] flax oil should never be used for cooking. When using flax oil, you should make sure it's cold-pressed, stored in a light-proof refrigerated container and use it up within a few weeks to prevent it from going rancid.

The rules above also apply to extra virgin olive oil, thus you should buy smaller, dark-colored bottles of olive oil that you know you can consume in about 2 weeks. Of course, during those 2 weeks you should store the oil bottle in a dark place.

And please, please, please, don't be fooled by bread or crackers labeled as "containing omega-3!"

You'll just spend your money for nothing. These products are cooked. The heat used to cook them adulterates omega-3. Companies selling cooked foods labeled as "containing omega-3", products like crackers or bread, should be fined for misleading consumers.

Sadly, the labeling laws are so vague, that manufacturers can claim pretty much whatever they feel to be an effective marketing hook for customers, without having to prove their claims.[242]

Just about any fish or seafood is a good source of natural omega-3 monounsaturated fats, but the fatter the fish, the higher the omega-3 content. However, such fish and seafood should not be overcooked or deep fried to enjoy the benefits of these fats. Deep frying and overcooking destroy all the omega-3 in such foods.[243] Smoked, salted and cured fish loses about half of its original omega-3 content. Raw fish and seafood would be the best choices when it comes to omega-3, but the possible health complications due to microbe contamination and rancidity require these foods to be cooked before eating.

Pregnant women, nursing women and young children should completely avoid shark, swordfish, tilefish, king mackerel, canned tuna, tuna steak and albacore, because of the high content of mercury.[244]

Mercury is found in water microorganisms, and small fish eat microorganisms, then big fish eat small fish. Large, long lived predatory fish, like sharks, swordfish, king mackerel and tilefish have more time to accumulate methyl mercury and are therefore the most toxic. Methyl mercury eaten by humans is almost completely absorbed from the digestive tract and accumulates in the brain, causing neurological damage and an increased risk of stroke. Damage to the brain of a developing fetus is more diffuse and widespread. Moreover, the fetal brain is sensitive to much lower doses of methyl mercury than the adult brain, so may be damaged even if the mother has no symptoms.[245] Long-term mercury accumulation in the brain and body can be a concern for anyone, but if we stay away from the large predatory fishes, we can enjoy the health benefits of fish intake.

For those of you still using their neurons in your brains, eating sufficient amounts of the right fats will help you go for hours without eating and without cravings. That is because food will taste better and blood sugar will remain stable for longer after a meal containing a normal level of healthy fats;[246] stable blood sugar and craving control are the keys to fat loss.

As I said earlier in this chapter, there is no proven connection between eating natural full-fat meat, eggs and milk products (such as butter, cheese and real yogurt) and heart diseases. Humans have thrived on animal fats for thousands of years. Animal fat is good for us. Of course, this would be true if the animal fat came from healthy animals. The real problem with most mass-produced animal products these days is that they come from animals given loads of antibiotics and fattened up with hormones.[247] The solution is to choose organically raised, grass-fed animal products.

A quick tip about eggs: when you buy eggs, they should have a number on them. The first figure of that number is 0, 1, 2 or 3. This rule applies in European Union countries. If you live outside EU, check your country specific regulations for the quality of eggs.

"Bio" eggs' numbers start with 0 and the unhealthiness of those eggs raises as the first figure of that number increases to 3. Bio eggs should come from free-range hens fed with grass and bio seeds. Eggs with numbers starting with 3 are cheaper, this is true. You can choose to eat fewer eggs and buy the expensive healthy ones.

- However, what do you think restaurants and cafeterias will buy to use in their egg-containing products, like birthday cakes, pastries or custard cookies?
- Think about it, ok?

Cutting back on fats to lose fat is a very bad idea

when it comes to effective fat loss.

- What are you going to eat?
- Are you going to follow food pyramids that encourage you to load your body with carbohydrates?

Then enjoy your insulin!

But, keep in mind that you will not touch one lipid droplet from your body as long as you're going to be insulin resistant.

CHAPTER 14: PROTEIN DIETS

- So what happens in your body when you don't eat carbs?
- Is this the weight loss solution you've been waiting for?
- And are you going to lose fat or are you going to lose weight?

Mainly, the human body uses glucose as fuel, when glucose is available. The main ways glucose can be obtained are:

1. eating carbohydrate food sources;
2. glycogenolysis: making glucose from liver glycogen or muscle glycogen; and
3. gluconeogenesis: making glucose from non-carbohydrate substrates such as proteins and glycerol, in the absence of dietary carbohydrates.

Glycogenolysis and gluconeogenesis are regulated by glucagon, the second pancreatic hormone involved in blood sugar regulation.[248]

The body's glycogen stores can provide glucose through glycogenolysis for about 6 hours. When blood sugar levels drop too low, glucagon turns off glycogenolysis and shuttles any left-over glycogenolytic intermediates to gluconeogenesis. Therefore, after the glycogen stores are depleted, glucose can be obtained through gluconeogenesis from dietary proteins or from the glycerol resulting from the breakdown of dietary or endogenous fats.

But as blood sugar rises, due to gluconeogenesis, the initial breakdown of body adipose fat is inhibited and de novo lipogenesis and muscle insulin resistance are stimulated.[249]

It is true that amino acids also stimulate insulin secretion, although to a far less extent than glucose, but the main problem protein rich diets have is that they stimulate glucagon secretion.[250] Due to glucagon, a high protein diet will make your body fat percentage increase, while the total body weight decreases due to muscle water loss.

You cannot just ban all carbs and lose fat by sticking to a too high-intake protein diets. This is just not how the human body works. As I explained in the Second Gear, to completely burn fatty acids, you need them inside 24h-contracting skeletal muscle cells with appropriate oxaloacetate storages. If you either eat too few carbohydrates, or if you secrete too much glucagon by eating too much protein, the result will be the same: incomplete fat burn, insulin resistance, muscle water loss, dehydration weight loss and increased body fat percentage.

All in all, as with the excess of any other nutrient, a protein intake that is too high stops fat loss and may cause fat gain through the insulin resistance pathway.

It is pretty certain that you will regain fat after stopping the protein diet due to the subsequent metabolic decrease. But, as incredible as it may seem, you even gain fat <u>during</u> the high protein diet. Please mind that I haven't wrote "weight gain", but "fat gain" – which happens during dehydration weight loss.

In the end, please remember that increasing the intake of dietary protein is important for fat loss,[251] but any "too much of a good thing is a bad thing."

CHAPTER 15: KETOGENIC DIETS

- Are ketogenic diets the solution to the worldwide obesity problem?

Many think so. Not me.

Some "doctors" mislead people into thinking that a good low-carb diet is a high fat diet, not a high protein diet. I have put the quotation marks around doctors, not because they are not real doctors, but because they don't act like ones. Doctors involved in the weight loss industry should remember the Hippocratic Oath. We are here to serve patients, not to mislead them for pecuniary reasons. The truth is that even though such "doctors" and many fitness gurus encourage people to go into ketosis to burn fat, this theory is just wrong biochemically.[252]

Let's just look for a moment at this "new" trend. The idea is still related to banning insulin from your system, but it also takes into account that dietary proteins stimulate insulin production. At a first glance, ketogenic diets are a bit smarter than proteic diets.

- But are they really?
- Should you eat a high fat, low carb, low proteic diet to become thin?
- And again, are you losing fat or are you losing weight?

The effectiveness of a very low carbohydrates and protein diet is supposedly based on the hypothesis that "When the body's glycogen stores are exhausted, the body starts utilizing fatty acids instead of glucose." With all due disrespect to people who have been through any medical school and still recommend such diets, humans don't break down fat stores when dietary fat intake is high.[253] You might choose to bypass this, because it calls your "miraculous idea" into question.

- But why would your body bother to break down fat stores when you feed it with a lot of fat?
- Would you empty your bank account if your monthly salary was high or huge?

My best bet is that you might save some of that money to increase your bank balance further.

I'm not even going to discuss the "what about the brain?" question, because your brain can use ketones to survive due to its reliance on a constant supply of oxaloacetate,[254] but due to the fatty acids-induced insulin resistance, those ketones will not come from the fat in your body, but from the fat in your food.[255] By using fatty acid derived ketones as energy sources, supplemented by the conversion of dietary proteins to glucose generated by glucagon, the body can maintain normal levels of blood glucose without dietary carbohydrates. This is true. But you will not burn body fat in the process.

You will function in survival mode. You will use dietary fatty acids and resulting ketones to stay alive. You will dehydrate yourself and lose water weight.[256] Your scales will be thrilled and so will you. But you will decrease your metabolism by emptying your muscle cells' glycogen one day at a time, because when supplied with fatty acids, muscle cells become insulin resistant, thus impermeable to glucose. Moreover, because of the huge stores of fatty acids inside muscle cells' mitochondria, some of these cells will be permanently damaged,[257] and if you'll have kids born after you did this to your muscles, they might even be born with muscles with less mitochondria.[258] Of course, that is only if you somehow manage to cure your insulin sensitivity enough to be fertile again, as insulin resistance is one of the main causes of infertility.[259, 260]

In conclusion, keep in mind that although insulin resistance, gluconeogenesis and ketosis have many downsides, they represent adaptive mechanisms during glucose shortage.

Please allow me to ask you two questions:

- Are these ketones you're measuring with expensive "ketones strips" coming from your fat body or are they really coming from the high fat foods you are eating during a ketogenic diet?

- And haven't you understood by now that the presence of ketones in your blood or urine equals stopped fat loss?[261]

You are a free person.

You can choose not to answer these questions.

You may choose not to care about their implications.

You may choose to live on a ketogenic diet for the rest of your life.

This is a choice, and it's your choice to take. I am not responsible for taking care of your body; you are. You think you are strong. You think your willpower will make a difference. You think you know best. Well... it's your body, so do as you please. Just remember that in order to lose fat we need to increase insulin sensitivity, and high fat diets just decrease it.[262]

I know a lot of lifelong athletes and fitness trainers think they function quite well on ketogenic diets. However, because of sports, such people have very high insulin sensitivity, and their cellular lipases

147

are upregulated by the everyday high intensity physical exercises they perform.[263] And also the high quantities of lactic acid that highly trained people develop during sports activities helps them to prevent not only insulin resistance in the muscles, but also ketosis, as lactic acid can be used in gluconeogenesis to create de novo glucose inside the liver despite a lowered carb intake. As I underlined above, these highly trained people just "think" they develop ketosis.[264] But their trained bodies are powerful enough on the inside to adapt to a temporarily lowered dietary glucose intake. Thus, applying their personal diets to sedentary, fat people is just wrong, because high fat diets just increases their insulin resistance further.

We need some carb intake to lose fat. And we need some protein intake to maintain fully active muscle mass. But the body is just not built to decrease adipose fat while fed with fat. This is biology, not common sense. Although we still have a lot to learn about fat loss, it's surely not based on wishful thinking.

And I don't even want to think about how hard it will be for these trainers or athletes not to become fat, in less than no time, when they lower their daily training level.[265]

Now let's consider some of the side effects of ketogenic diets. Yes **diets – just like medication or**

supplements – do have side effects. And you should be fully informed and accept the risk of suffering from such side effects before starting any diet plan.

Though ketosis on its own is not necessarily dangerous, prolonged ketosis **does** lead to ketoacidosis, even in the healthiest people. However, most people follow high fat diets only for short periods of time, so they usually don't get that far. I cannot tell you how fast or how slowly your body will enter ketoacidosis if you continue a ketogenic diet for longer than a few days. However when your muscle cells' oxaloacetate supply is finished and you keep depositing fatty acids inside your muscle cells' mitochondria, that will be the starting point of your diet slavery. Remember that!

Mild ketosis side effects include bad breath and abdominal gas. If you continue with the ketogenic diet for more than a few days you will experience weakness, nausea and dizziness. If you really keep going and live in a state of ketosis for a longer time, you just cannot avoid ketoacidosis and its side effects, which include:

1. fatigue and lethargy: due to muscle mitochondria breakage;
2. diarrhea or constipation: due to the low intake of dietary fiber;
3. depression: due to a deficient intake of vitamins

and minerals;

4. liver damage: due to fatty acids being deposited inside the liver cells;

5. kidney damage: due to damaging nephrons' membranes and messing with the acidic-basic pH of the blood;

6. bone structure damage: due to the fact that when the pH of the blood becomes acidic, the body uses calcium to neutralize this;

7. and, in extreme cases, death.

Let me give you one more piece of bad news. Not only during ketoacidosis does blood become too acidic. Blood pH lowers even after a "habitual" binge eating episode based on proteins and fats.[266]

- You might ask yourself, who the heck binges on proteins and fats?

Well, despite the low appetite associated with such diets, many followers of low-carb diets eventually do so. Add caffeine and artificial sweeteners contained in diet drinks to glue your day together, and you might as well accept osteoporosis as a very real part of your live.[267]

No, you will not develop osteoporosis overnight. But you will use calcium to normalize the blood pH, and you will take that calcium from your bones. That is not even to mention that proteic and ketogenic diets are low on calcium intake anyway.

- Again, why would you do this to your body?

- Why would you endanger your health?
- And how would you act if you witnessed another person forcing someone to live like this?
- Do you think that "forcing others" doesn't apply to forcing yourself?
- You are forcing your body to survive your unhealthy ideas. Isn't it the same?

Up to a point, it isn't. Because these popular, highly marketed diets are based on theoretical guesses and defended by biased trials. The weight loss world is in chaos, because too many nutritionists and doctors continue to parrot outdated misinformation to make a fast buck.

You just need to open your eyes and stop paying for these people's salaries with your hard earned money and with your health. Or not.

CHAPTER 16: GLYCEMIC INDEX DIETS

All these theories about proteic diets and Glycemic Index (GI) or Glycemic Load (GL) diets are actually quite old.[268] And despite the fact that a lot of people have put their trust in them as being smart new findings, they have failed dieters since the 80's.

In reality, low-carb diets can also be low-GL/low GI diets and vice versa, depending on the intake of carbohydrates in a particular diet. All I can agree with is that there is a little more scientific research that supports the low GL index diets.

Proteic diets treat all carbs as having the same effect on metabolism, based on the assumption that all carbohydrates have the same effect on metabolism. This is, at least, lazy thinking. Providing a higher level of honesty, low GL diets are based on the laboratory-measured changes in blood glucose levels caused by the intake of various carbohydrates.

But those changes are particular, not general. You cannot just generalize the glycemic effect a food might have either eaten alone, or eaten in specific combinations.[269] It is hilarious to think that you can in any way estimate the glycemic effect a meal will have, even for the same human on different days or at different stages of hunger. For instance scientists found a GI variation of 17.8% between 23 healthy adults eating the same quantity of the same bread and **a GI variation of 42.8% for the same person eating the same quantity of bread, on different days.**[270] A scientifically proven GI variation of 42% is more than significant, from my point of view.

And please allow me to tell you, if you don't at least suspect this by now, that these measurements are done on standard blood sugar. In reality, blood sugar varies during the day in all individuals, thus eating a particular food starting on a higher or lower blood sugar has different metabolic effects than eating that food on a set blood sugar. Therefore, to generalize, to create scientific charts of GI or GL foods, and to recommend them as guidelines for weight loss is just abusive and deceptive, potentially undermining the trust people have in the medical world.

Moreover, any food preparation influences the GI or GL of the meal.[271] Grinding or cooking will almost always elevate these indexes, because the food becomes easier to digest.

And we mainly consume combinations of foods. The addition of other foods that contain fiber, proteins or fats generally modifies the glycemic effect of a whole meal, making it higher or lower in a way most scientists know to be impossible to predict. Even calculating the GL of a mixed meal based on the GLs of the individual ingredients, has **an accuracy of no more than 58%.**[272] This is because the total <u>percentage</u> of carbohydrates within any mixed meal is different than the predicted amount, leaving us with nothing more than a wild guess about the glycemic effect that particular meal might have.[273] Furthermore, some foods cause a disproportionate glycemic response relative to their carbohydrate load. For instance, foods like pizza create a significantly higher glycemic response than the simple weighed average of the ingredient GI's would predict. The reality is that fiber, proteins and fats influence the absorption of glucose from carbohydrates eaten at the same time. And each food out there contains different amounts of carbohydrates, proteins and fats.

When you're eating complete meals, containing carbohydrates, fats and proteins, you have a lower insulin response than when you eat carbohydrates alone.[274]

And a lower insulin response after eating is the start of fat loss.

Also, some carbohydrates are indigestible to humans and some require grinding and cooking to become absorbable through the intestinal wall. And not all the carbohydrates from a food pass into our blood after we eat it. We cannot even predict the amount of carbohydrates we might absorb after eating an apple, as it can differ based upon how ripe or how raw that apple is.

The presence or absence of hunger, the amount of food we eat, with what other foods we combine it, how much that food is processed and even how that food is cooked, are all factors that influence the glycemic response. Because foods influence digestion in such complex ways, it is impossible to predict the glycemic effect of a particular meal in a particular person on a particular day. No matter how vigorously the GI or GL diets are marketed these days, the basis of such diets is merely self-awareness.

GI or GL are just numbers in a chart that provides **a hypothetical idea** about the food impact on blood sugar level and possible insulin related problems.[275]

The low-insulin index diet was the scientists' next "smart" idea. But measuring the amount of insulin in the blood after a meal rather than measuring the amount of glucose is just as misleading. You, or anyone else for that matter, cannot predict how much of a particular nutrient from a food will be absorbed into the blood after one eats that food or what the glycemic or insulimic response to that food will be.[276]

Predicting glucose blood level or insulin blood level after eating any particular food relies purely on guesswork. And guesswork is not something that scientists should offer to the general public as guidelines. Scientists are wasting their time and people are becoming fatter and fatter.

CHAPTER 17: FOOD COMBINATIONS

I hope that thus far, you have understood my point:

To lose fat, you need to eat carbohydrates, proteins and fats at every meal, to ensure you have a lower postprandial amount of insulin in the blood.

Eating complete meals when hungry (thus starting to eat when the blood sugar is low enough to activate the hypothalamic hunger center), has these beneficial effects for fat loss:

1. it keeps muscle membranes permeable for glucose;

2. it keeps the enzymes that regulate fat-burn up and running;

3. it keeps us satiated for longer periods of times between meals; and

4. it enhances the eating pleasure derived from

eating natural, whole foods that taste better.

However, many people were "educated" by popular weight loss "gurus" to think that combining carbohydrates with proteins and/ or fats somehow messes with digestion, because supposedly the stomach is not able to digest them all together at the same time.

Well, ladies and gentlemen, introducing: Digestion Physiology 1:1!!! Please pay attention, Google "carbohydrate digestion", or at least search for these words on Wikipedia.

-   So, are you with me?
1. Digestion is only the first step in the transformation of food into nutrients usable by our cells. We also need intestinal absorption for nutrients to be able to enter our blood to be transported to cells for use.
2. Digestion mainly happens in the small intestine, **not in the stomach.**[277]
3. Cooked carbohydrate digestion barely starts in the mouth, due to the enzyme called "salivary amylase", but it stops in the stomach regardless of the presence or absence of fats or proteins.[278]
4. And although it is true that gastric acid deactivates salivary amylase inside the stomach, the pancreatic amylase released in the small intestine is so powerful that it can perform the carbohydrate digestion entirely on its own, with

or without the preliminary help of the salivary amylase.[279]

5. Separating fruits from main meals is an idea based on the supposition that the fiber within the fruits somehow impedes stomach digestion and "traps" food inside the stomach, causing putrefaction and fermentation.

6. However, fiber from fresh fruits isn't any different than fiber from fresh vegetables.

    -   Why would the fiber from fresh vegetables be OK combined with meat (just an example), but the fiber from fruits not OK?

    Fiber is fiber, and the facts that it's important to remember are: that we mostly do not digest it at all and that it is very beneficial for the digestion of all nutrients, be they proteins, fats or carbohydrates.

7. Also, the putrefaction and fermentation of food does not happen in the stomach, but in the large intestine, if you have eaten too much food high in fiber,[280] or if the eaten food has not been kept long enough in the stomach[281] or has been released too quickly or in bigger quantities than the digestive enzymes within the small intestine are able to work on.

These weird ideas that nutrient digestion is more effective when food spends less time in the stomach than it biologically would need to, or that the digestion of nutrients happens in the stomach, are just making people have meals that are too high in carbohydrates, imbalanced meals that may be the root cause of fattening due to the subsequent muscle insulin resistance.[282]

8. Also, the fact that fiber in a mixed meal (either from fruits, vegetables or cooked starches) increases the time the food spends in the stomach **is a good thing**! You should aim for it at each meal, because a longer gastric stay allows enough time for the intestinal juices to be secreted and discharged into the small intestine by the pancreas, bile and intestine. It also has the potential to generate a better postprandial blood sugar level.[283]

   - Why the heck would anyone avoid these beneficial effects that fiber has by eating fruits outside of meals or by separating carbohydrate containing meals from protein and fat containing foods?

Such eating behavior will only spell irritable bowel syndrome on their foreheads.

So, please remember: it is not the stomach that mainly digests the food we eat, but the small intestine. The stomach is only a warehouse where the eaten food is properly blended and stored to allow the much needed time for the secretion of intestinal juices.

Moreover, the fiber within a fruit has no

different metabolic effect when combined with meat than the fiber within vegetables.[284] This is just a supposition made by people who have never taken a physiology class in their lives. And, as I said, don't take my word for it and also don't bury your head in anecdotal evidence. To successfully achieve fat loss, it is extremely important to be objective and search and see for yourself!

As with any other carbohydrates, eating fruits outside meals, as snacks or as fruit meals, will create a higher increase in blood sugar and insulin levels and impede your fat loss, because of the potential subsequent insulin resistance. So don't consider fruits as some special nutrient source that impedes digestion of other nutrients. When you want to eat fruits, eat them as part of complete meals, as they do not impede other nutrients' digestion in any way.[285]

It is of the highest importance to always try your best to eat all nutrients (proteins, carbohydrates and fats together) when hungry, in order to feel more satiated and have a steadier blood sugar for longer after the meal.[286]

Please note that because fat is actually associated with protein and carbohydrates in real whole foods, I will only speak about combining proteins and carbohydrates, implying the presence of fat in the combination.

Essential amino acids are amino acids that are

mandatory for health, which our body cannot produce. Thus, we must "eat" them. Proteins from vegetal foods are not complete when it comes to the essential (for humans) amino acids they can provide. Proteins from animal foods contain the complete number of essential amino acids humans need in order to be healthy. So, I consider animal foods (like meat, fish, milk, cheese, yoghurt, eggs and any other products that we can eat from animals) as the best protein food sources we can eat as humans.

With all due respect to vegetarians out there, plant foods are mostly sources of carbohydrates. The proteic content of most plant foods is low and the quality of their proteins is even lower. If you are a vegetarian, please do not be offended! When talking about the "quality" of the plant proteins I'm not saying that animal proteins are in any way better or worse. What I'm saying is that plant proteins are of lower quality for humans, because they do not provide all the essential amino acids unless carefully combined. Yes, there are some plant foods that contain more and better proteins than others. But the constant focus on combining them correctly so as not to endanger health induces food preoccupation faster than anything else.

Losing fat while vegetarian is damn hard, because the optimum protein intake is harder to achieve.[287] Being vegetarian and fit really proves you have willpower, but up to a point it takes your focus off other things you can do with your life besides eating. But I must admit that vegetarianism sounds far better than the Western Diet full of trans fat foods, GMO meats full of antibiotics and growth hormones and other "modern era foods" many people eat on the run.

However, I think the best nutritional outcome can only come from combining proteins and carbohydrates at every meal. Thus, I consider eating in the Third Gear as eating animal and vegetal foods together.

- Simplified thinking, right?

Poor long-term adherence to diets is a crucial issue for overweight and obese people.[288] Weight loss through dieting and exercise tends to be successful for the first 6 months, but in the long-term most individuals are unable to maintain this weight loss; fat loss rules **must be kept simple** in order to increase long-term adherence.[289]

And I'm not only trying to keep it simple. I'm also trying to get rid of all the food preoccupation, not to say obsession, which diets can lead to.[290]

So, I urge you to stop thinking about consuming equal quantities of both proteins and carbohydrates, or about any quantities, for that matter. And I'm not saying you can eat the whole fridge when you're hungry either. But even you cannot establish beforehand the amount of food "you're allowed" to eat when you're hungry.

-   How would you know beforehand how many nutrients your body has used since your last meal and how many will be enough to cover the current needs of your body?

You must dive into your body and you must listen its true – there is no other way.

Although highly promoted as a weight loss tool, estimating your body's needs can be inaccurate enough to generate or aggravate insulin resistance, causing the body fat percentage to increase even in the thinner looking people who do not obey the hunger and satiation body guidelines.[291]. Think of food when you get hungry, not before or after.[292]

Use your mind to conquer the world, not to control your body! The physiology of the human body is so complex that God decided the conscious mind isn't reliable enough for taking care of survival. Speaking about it might make a lot of people look smart, but it won't make a difference to who your internal boss is. You are not in control of your body and you never will be. The more you focus on weight loss, the more you'll just put your life on hold and become fatter.[293] So, focus on hunger and satiation, not on maddening diets.

If we consider animal foods as sources of protein and plant foods as sources of carbohydrates, eating them together is the only thing you need to ensure you do to speed up the fat loss process. The percentage of each in the whole meal is irrelevant, don't think about it! Focus on building your meals around whole foods, full of essential amino acids and fatty acids, fiber and carbohydrates that are naturally "contained" and not "added" to foods. Think only about the quality of food and allow your hypothalamus to guide you through satiation about how much or how little you need to eat at each meal.

Also don't beat your head about which natural foods contains carbs, which carbs are better than others or any other fancy dieting ideas. The fact that is a natural whole food is enough.

-   Do you need to know advanced mechanics to shift gears and drive your car in the city?

Achieving carbohydrate and protein intake at the same time is the most efficient fat loss related decision we can make at any meal. Combining animal and plant foods will provide you with all the nutrients you need and with a steady blood sugar level for a longer period of time after the meal, both of which are essential for fat loss. You will also enjoy a greater sensation of satiation due to the proteins and fats from the animal foods, and better health protection due to the vitamins, minerals and fibers contained in the plant foods.

It takes a little exercise to learn the technique.

But it is only going to be as hard as learning how to drive. With practice, you will enjoy the freedom of eating the food you like when you're hungry and stopping, without guilt, when you're full. So, be positive, patient and persistent in practicing this!

Working out for 30 minutes a day, every other day, whilst also eating animal food sources and plant food sources together, when and for as long we are hungry is enough to achieve a steady long term fat loss.

But the miracle seekers of the diet world have messed with even this basic principle of human physiology.

They say that combining proteins and carbohydrates makes people gain weight, because the carbohydrates are digested in the mouth (they say, not me) and the proteins are digested in the stomach. Apparently, this distinction between the locations at which the respective groups of nutrients are supposedly being digested is the root of our worldwide obesity problem. They say you can eat whatever you wish and as much as you wish, as long as you are not combining proteins with carbohydrates.[294]

This absurd idea was actually born in the head of a doctor! Doctor Howard Hay developed this "eating method" in the 1930s. Dr. Hay's assumptions have been discussed controversially since he first published them. Because his hypothesis cannot be proven (there is absolutely no scientific proof of any sort to support this "idea") or disproven in a mentally sane way, its followers think it must be right. None of these miracle seekers were thinking of hunger, biochemistry, human physiology or anything of the sort. It's like saying obesity is caused by the fact that your nose is not your leg. Now prove to the crazy person that his nose is not his leg!

Please don't consider the time you spend feeding yourself as spare time to catch up with anything you've been meaning to get around to. Consider the time you need to feed yourself as an important time you should use to take care of your own body. Consider it a priority, not a waste of time! Eat slowly, chew your food well and don't do any other activity – while eating, just eat. No reading your emails, working, watching TV, or anything else that it ever occurs to you to do while eating.

Also, try to eat at a table or at least sitting down somewhere, even when eating on the street or at a barbeque party. Focus on the taste and texture of the food you're eating. If you were really hungry before eating, and if now you're fully savoring a complete meal constituted of animal plant foods, you will be able to feel satiation.

And of course, there will be times when you just want a cup of warm milk, a piece of fruit or an ice cream. If you think it's important, slow down your fat loss speed and eat them in the Second or the First Gear, or completely without hunger with your fat burning engine stopped. No blaming or regrets required.[295] Enjoy them and then continue along your road.

Use your brain to conquer the world, not to obsess over food and weight loss – that's your hypothalamus's job. And remember: success begins at the edge of your comfort zone. So, just let go of this continuous weight loss struggle & trust in your body to guide you to your healthy weight. It will!

Third Gear Recap:

Small-step goal no. 1: **Eat only when and only for as long as you are biologically hungry.**

Never eat food you dislike. *

Sleep enough. *

Small-step goal no. 2: **Do 30minutes of cardio/ anaerobic exercises every other day.**

Don't use any electrical weight loss procedure. *

Small-step goal no. 3: **Eat both vegetal and animal foods when hungry.** (Please do not start to work on achieving this goal before mastering and practicing the first two goals on a daily basis, for at least 1 full week.)

After successfully achieving goal no. 3 on a daily basis for more than 1 week, you end the Preparation stage of your Changing Progress and can drive further on the road that will lead you towards the thinnest and healthiest body you can biologically have.

* These are not mandatory goals, but they might sabotage your fat loss unless taken into consideration.

Fourth Gear

Small-step goal no. 4: **Hydrate yourself with at least 1 liter of water every day.**

This one is harder, but it might actually speed up your fat loss a lot by decreasing "artificial" hunger caused by dehydration. Also, if you've taken your time learning to control your "car" in the Third Gear, driving your body in the Fourth Gear is really low on emotional fuel consumption. From hot summer days to Christmas holidays, driving in the Fourth Gear will give you the gorgeous body you always dreamt to have.

In the Fourth Gear, you cannot have more than one regular coffee per day, and that means regular for you. If you like to drink your coffee with milk and sugar, go for it. Just keep it to one cup per day.

You must also limit your alcohol intake to one drink per day.

You cannot drink any sweetened drinks, either with sugar or with artificial sweeteners.

And don't drink sports drinks unless you're an athlete.

CHAPTER 18: HYDRATION

I estimate that a lot of people will be surprised by the fact that I put hydration higher than food combinations, when it comes to fat loss. I have a lot of reasons for doing this, but the main reason is:

Too many people eat and drink unhealthy, addictive foods and drinks, because of cellular dehydration (read thirst).

- "What??"

Yes, sadly this is true.

I am actually not talking about the dietary fluid intake per se, but specifically about drinking water. While it is true that an overly high fluid intake can temporarily decrease appetite, a real physical need for hydration (osmotic thirst) will increase the appetite for salty foods and drinks.[296] Eating out of thirst or out of being cold (I talked about eating out of being cold in the Second Gear) induces the same anabolic reactions as overeating, because, in such a situation,

171

the hypothalamic hunger center is stimulated by the irradiated wave sent by a nearby overstimulated nervous center, not by blood sugar.

Another reason I put hydration above food combinations is that a lot of people on diets just replace eating with drinking coffee or diet drinks.[297] These soft drinks, with or without sugar, can increase both insulin resistance and appetite.[298] So, good bye, fat loss!

Water is not the panacea for every disease, but it has the power to make us feel and be healthy. Being one of the main constituents of our bodies, water helps regulate all our systems. So, you must agree that drinking water is one important healthy habit.

-    But what has water to do with fat loss?

A lot!

If you drink more than one coffee per day and a lot of soda, diet drinks, alcohol or even too much fruit juice or tea, you will really dehydrate your body, both because you will not feel thirsty for water anymore and because such drinks are dehydrating per se. Reducing your intake of "other drinks" and increasing your water intake is a must for fat loss, because all these "other drinks," besides artificially inducing hunger, also indirectly deregulate insulin secretion and cause a myriad of metabolic disturbances.[299]

Caffeine containing drinks (coffee, tea, soft

drinks) and alcoholic drinks are diuretics, which means they stimulate urination.[300] So, if it is not enough that these drinks don't hydrate the body, they also increase dehydration even further by robbing the body of the little water it still has.

Let's take a quick look at sports drinks. While water alone rehydrates the body, the water, electrolytes and carbohydrates found in sports drinks rehydrate the body much faster. But this "much faster" factor is important only for competition athletes or when you're participating in a long endurance aerobic exercise like cycling. Although sports drinks can be beneficial to athletes looking to replenish lost fluids and glycogen stores quickly, they should never be consumed by inactive individuals or by people who engage in just moderate exercise.[301] Water is enough for these last categories of people.

Another aspect is that many people do not consider drinks as food and, therefore, they may gain weight due to the excessive carbohydrate intake caused by consuming these drinks.[302] This fact is extremely important in the case of sports drinks, which have an even higher carbohydrate content meant to replenish the glycogen stores of a highly active muscle and not to increase the fat stores! Thus, if you are not a busy trainer or an athlete, you should never consume sports drinks.

Another fluid people drink instead of water is

fruit juice. But even fruit juices squeezed from fresh fruits just before drinking are high in fructose. Many people think that fructose is not as "unhealthy" as sugar. However, the only reason why fructose is not absorbed as fast as sugar is due to fruit's fiber: fiber which is removed when you make the juice. Another problem is that an excessive fructose intake (such as that which happens when consuming drinks containing high fructose corn syrup) will be directly transformed into fat by the liver.[303]   In addition, sweetened drinks high in fructose and either glucose or artificial sweeteners may induce insulin resistance of both muscle <u>and</u> adipose tissue, consequently generating dyslipidemia.[304] So, drink fruit juices as rarely as you can, because, although healthier than most other soft drinks, they can contribute to fattening too. Eating whole fruits is a much better choice both for your health and for fat loss. And for your teeth, a dentist might add.[305]

Most people postpone drinking until they feel thirsty, but, by this point the body might be already dehydrated.[306] Dehydration is a problem that can only be prevented or solved through consciously making the effort to drink enough water and through limiting your intake of "other drinks."

The main "reasons" that some people don't drink enough water are:

1. they don't feel thirsty;

2. they don't like the taste of water; and that
3. they forget to drink it.

Such people might start their day with a nice coffee, drink iced teas or soft drinks all day long, and finish the day with one or more glasses of wine or beer. Whenever you say to yourself that you don't have time to drink water, remember that it only takes a few seconds to drink a glass of water, but the effects of proper hydration are long-term miracles for your health and fat loss. I cannot imagine why anyone would treat themselves so badly! There is no difference between a slave and such a person.

- Are you a slave or a free person that can permit himself the "luxury" of drinking some water?

It is easy to knock out the excuse "I don't feel thirsty". You might become dehydrated if you wait to feel thirsty before drinking your water. Therefore, waiting to feel thirst is just a big mistake. So, don't wait to feel thirst, just make a habit of drinking a glass of water every one or two hours. That's it! And if you don't like the taste of water, join the slim top models "still water and lemon" club. Or get creative and brainstorm some new ideas that can help you enjoy your water.

The excuse of forgetting to drink is just childish.

- Do you ever forget to drink your coffee, do you forget to buy and carry your soft drink bottle, or do you forget your beer?

- Or what about your car, do you forget to refill your tank?

C'mon!

I cannot believe my ears when I hear about people using only the best gasoline and car oils for their cars and only junk food, coffee, soft drinks and alcoholic drinks for their own body.

CHAPTER 19: CAFFEINE AND FAT LOSS

The main issues relating to caffeine and fat loss are insulin resistance and dehydration.[307, 308]

Caffeine and artificial sweeteners don't increase blood sugar and insulin secretion directly, but indirectly by increasing muscle cells' insulin resistance.[309] As I explained you, this is very bad news for your fat loss!

Drink it many times a day with sugar or artificial sweeteners and you might as well tattoo "insulin resistant" on your forehead. One or two cups of caffeine containing drinks associated with hunger and drunk with food should be fine, but more than that or drinking them without food will just make you a bit fatter every day.

Now, a lot of people think that caffeine is brown.

It isn't.[310]

Caffeine is crystal clear and it is used as a food preservative in most soft drinks, carbonated or not.[311] So, cola and coffee aren't the only drinks containing caffeine.[312] Most soft drinks contain caffeine, thus potentially decreasing insulin sensitivity. Therefore, you should avoid any soft drinks. And by all means possible, avoid artificially sweetened, "diet" sodas!

Artificial sweeteners are just a scientists' bad joke.

They were invented to permit diabetics to enjoy the sweet taste, despite their disease. But the sour truth is that they deregulate insulin secretion to a greater extent than sugar.[313] You might think drinking diet sodas or replacing sugar in your coffee with saccharine or stevia will help you lose weight or at least maintain your weight. Think again!

The only "benefit" such sweeteners have is caloric content. And if you still worry about caloric content, you might as well close this book right now, because you are wasting your time reading human physiology principles you are not able or willing to understand.

I don't care about the "popularity" of calories. Calories are just a tool the weight loss industry uses to blame and dismiss fat people. Focusing on calories and not on the actual mechanisms behind the fattening process is going to keep you and your children their slaves for life.

CHAPTER 20: ALCOHOL AND FAT LOSS

-   Can you drink alcohol and lose fat?

Yes.[314]

And No.[315]

The line between the "Yes" and the "No" is fairly fluid. Just keep in mind that alcohol is a "sugar." Sugar equals insulin. And excess sugars of any kind equal insulin resistance and subsequent fat gain.

-   Am I saying not to eat sugar?

No.

-   Am I saying not to drink alcohol?

No.

I'm saying that when driving in the Fourth Gear, if you want to drink alcohol, have one drink per day at the same time as eating food, while hungry, to keep your blood sugar and postprandial insulin secretion under control.[316]

One "drink" is considered to be 12 ounces of beer, 5 ounces of wine or 1 ½ ounces of spirits; in other words any quantity that provides about 10-12 grams of alcohol. On the label of any alcoholic drink bottle you can find the alcoholic content of that drink. If you have a hard time understanding what "one drink" means, then here is your rule:

Drink only as much as you can while still being able to legally drive a car.

- How much can you drink so that if a cop stopped you, you would not get into trouble?

Moderate drinking means that we should not exceed one alcoholic drink defined as above.

But don't fall into the trap of thinking that you must consume some alcohol, because it induces "health benefits." If you're slim, you do some regular sport or even walk your dog daily at a fast pace, you don't smoke, and you eat a generally healthy diet, drinking alcohol won't add that much to your health. If you don't drink, there is no need to start.

But if you like to enjoy your favorite drink from time to time, just make sure you don't overdo it and try to make the best of your pleasure. Sit down, don't hurry, and savor every drop of your drink (with your best friends or loved ones, if possible). Also, don't consume your "alcoholic allowance" for one week during just one night of drinking. Drinking binges can be extremely dangerous for your health.[317]

So, in the Fourth Gear, you should limit your alcoholic intake to one drink per day, and drink it with meals to slow down alcohol absorption.

Scientists think that most people underestimate their alcohol intake.[318] So, as with hunger, you can keep a log for a week. Write down, daily, all the drinks you've had. This should shed some light on your drinking habits.

If you have trouble restricting yourself to moderate drinking, don't start. And if you do start, try to make a conscious effort to stay within the limits of a preset "drinking budget."

Don't drink alone or if you're unhappy.

Eat before or with every drink you have.

Don't exceed the daily maximum.

When going out, also drink water, fruit juice, coffee or tea. Alcoholic drinks are not the only options and never think they are mandatory in social situations.

Moreover, don't fool yourself into thinking that if you mix alcohol with other beverages, it won't add up. The rum in the cola will go straight to your blood with or without the cola.[319]

Also, remember to look your best whenever you over-drink, because only the beauty of others increases with the number of beers.

In moderation, alcohol increases good HDL-cholesterol,[320] and decreases bad LDL-cholesterol.[321]

Therefore it can have health benefits like a lower risk of heart attack and stroke, Alzheimer's or dementia. But any benefit is just washed away by the consumption of large doses, which will, at the very least, result in drunkenness, followed by a hangover, despite any hydration measures applied after heavy drinking.

In relation to fat loss, alcoholic drinks are just another source of carbohydrates. Alcohol has the potential to generate hyperglycemia, excessive insulin secretion and subsequent hypoglycemia. But if you don't overdo it and if you associate drinking with eating, the total postprandial blood sugar will stay within a healthy range. Every time you consume any carbohydrates, including alcohol or sweetened drinks, with complete meals containing proteins from animal foods and fibers from vegetal foods, you will have a lower postprandial insulin response.[322]

So, never overdo it with alcohol and never drink it without eating.

Good sense should always prevail when it comes to any drink you consume!

CHAPTER 21: TEAS AND WEIGHT LOSS

Many pharmaceutical products were originally derived from plant sources, thus herbs may be effective remedies for medical conditions. But the lack of information regarding the side effects of herbal remedies creates the false idea that herbal remedies don't have any. The general public sees herbal remedies as a natural and safer alternative to medication. But don't be fooled: if we don't know that much about their harmful effects, it does not mean they are safe(r). And although scientists can be a little arrogant when it comes to herbal remedies, we should always trust pharmaceutical products before herbal remedies because:

1. herbal remedies require no peer reviewed testing with regard to their safety, purity or efficacy;

2. and there is no legal requirement for post

marketing surveillance.[323]

Beside impurities, adulterants and herb misidentifications, plants contain complex mixtures of chemicals. But herbal remedies are not tested for interactions, either between the chemicals contained in one plant and chemicals from other plants within the same herbal remedy,[324] or between these plants' chemicals and prescribed medication.[325]

For instance, ginkgo biloba may increase the risk of hemorrhage, and it interacts with aspirin-type medication (NSAIDs). Also, some chemicals contained by ginseng inhibit coagulation in vitro and prolong coagulation times in animal studies. Thus, the intake of such remedies should be discontinued before any surgery and reported to the doctors.[326]

Moreover, there are no internationally recognized names for most plants. There are many confusing synonyms, meaning the name of some plants can be archaic or different depending upon geographical region. In addition, the concentration of active ingredients in plants varies depending on the harvested part of the plant, on the plant's maturity at the time of the harvest, on the time of year the harvest is performed, on geography and soil conditions, and on soil composition and contaminants.[327]

Therefore, the real dose of an active compound in an herbal remedy is impossible to predict.

You should not associate "natural" with "safe." Opium and marijuana are "natural" too!

In my opinion, herbal remedies should be subjected to the same examination as traditional pharmaceutical medicines, which include checking for biological plausibility, consistency of research results, dose-response effects, reproducibility of the research in different contexts using different methodologies and a correct temporality between cause and effect. Until herbal remedies are put through that kind of testing, their safety, quality and efficacy cannot be guaranteed.

- Now, regarding weight loss teas: all I can say is what are you trying to lose?

Because what such teas are actually doing is dehydrating the body.[328]

- **Do you want to lose weight or do you want to lose fat?**

Many fat people don't really care what they lose, as long as they lose... something. Just for such people: please carefully read again the chapter on Hydration!

CHAPTER 22: LIQUID DIETS

Liquid diets have been around for at least three decades.

- Are they the miracle diets you've been waiting for?
- And what's so miraculous about them?

Despite the fact that many celebrities swear by them, liquid diets are just short-term, very low calorie diets.[329]

- So is anything miraculous about a very low calorie diet?

I don't think so!

- Remember the vow "I will not use any of my neurons until I lose weight"?

Well, you should go to a real church and place your hand on a bible to make that vow in front of God before starting a liquid diet. This way you can be really honest about the intention of leaving your body for the duration of the diet. Except that, sadly, you cannot get out of your body. So, you'll be deep within it when sluggishness, fatigue and dizziness hit you – hard.

Nevertheless, the effects of any diet will last only for as long as you are on that diet and, at most, it will take an equal amount of time to become as fat as you were before the diet, once you quit.[330] So, this is the question you should ask yourself before even considering such a diet:

- **How long do you think you can live on a liquid diet?[331]**

You must ask yourself this question before starting a liquid diet, because long time liquid diets can damage your intestinal tract, your liver and gallbladder, your kidneys, your heart and your immune system. And they can kill you![332]

- Will you lose weight?
Yes.
- Will you lose fat?
No. Not even one gram.[333]

As I've explained in the Third Gear, the human body's survival response to very low calorie diets is insulin resistance in muscle cells and fat storage. You'll only dehydrate yourself and decrease your metabolism during such a diet. Not only that, but you will also have a hard time keeping the weight off after such a diet.[334] The nutrient intake of liquid diets is so low that as soon as the "Hell" is over, the weight gain

187

will follow, no matter how careful you are with your after-diet-eating.

This means that, no matter what you eat after a liquid diet, you will become fatter than before the diet by eating less than you used to.[335]

"Five percent of people think. Ten percent of people think they think. And the other eighty five percent would sooner die than think."

- Thomas Edison

I feel compassion for desperate people. And if you desperately want or need to lose fat, then just run away, as far as you can, from liquid diets.

The truth is that very low calorie diets and liquid diets are fattening diets.[336] They should be recommended only for skinny people trying to gain fat. As soon as you get this into your head, you'll get out of the diet industry payers' club and start losing fat for a change.

Fourth Gear Recap:

Small-step goal no. 1:_**Eat only when and only for as long as you are biologically hungry.**

Never eat food you dislike *

Sleep enough *

Small-step goal no. 2: **Do 30minutes of cardio/ anaerobic exercises every other day.**

Don't use any electrical weight loss procedure *

Small-step goal no. 3: **Eat both vegetal and animal foods when hungry.**

Small step goal no. 4: **Hydrate yourself with at least 1 liter of water every day.** (Please do not start to work on achieving this goal until mastering and practicing the first 3 ones for at least 1 week!)

Limit yourself to one coffee and one alcoholic drink/ day *

Don't drink soft drinks or weight loss teas *

* These are not mandatory goals, but they might sabotage your fat loss unless taken into consideration.

189

Fifth Gear

Small-step goal no. 5: **Do 30 minutes of interval cardio training/ or 30 minutes of anaerobic exercises every day.**

Small-step goal no. 6: **Eat only healthy foods.**

Driving in the Fifth Gear requires an advanced state of awareness and self care. The fast lane of the freeway should only be driven by those powerful enough to take on the challenges that come along with the Top Gears. It is harder to stop and you could end up crashed or even killed if you don't master your driving skills. It is high on emotional "fuel" consumption; however, it will get to your dream body destination you faster than ever.

Cardio interval training is highly effective and when alternated with anaerobic exercise it will do wonders for your insulin sensitivity.

Expel man-made foods and eat a high variety of fresh nature-made foods. Educate yourself about the science behind healthy eating.

Keep in mind that when it comes to losing fat, as much as when it comes to driving, you must be in control or you'll crash!

CHAPTER 23: INTERVAL TRAINING

I have spoken in the Second Gear about the wonders that anaerobic exercises can do for your metabolism and about how to eat after a workout. I will not repeat myself. Just read the Second Gear again if you need to. What is new in the Fifth Gear is that you must exercise every day and that you must replace casual cardio exercises with the highly effective cardio interval training.

There is no need to increase the duration of the exercise from 30 minutes per day. I'm not saying that you cannot do sport for more than 30 minutes; just that you don't need to. You can do high intensity interval training exercises for as long as you wish. As always, you're in the driver's seat. You get to decide what best suit your own body.

But, keep in mind that long periods of cardio endurance training is not as effective in terms of fat loss as short periods of cardio interval training,[337] and that sport can also make you ravenously hungry.[338]

30 minutes of intense cardio interval training is an amazingly beneficial time-saving strategy,[339] as effective as 60 minutes of moderate endurance training in improving your health, fitness and metabolism.[340] So, it can be a training strategy easier to fit in a busy daily schedule. And don't let yourself be fooled, a full hour of moderate intensity sport today won't mean that tomorrow you'll get a free day if you wish to drive in the Fifth Gear.

To drive in the Fifth Gear to fat loss, you must exercise **every** day. Slow down to lower Gears if you don't have those 30 minutes to exercise. This is a choice. And fat loss is a choice you have to make every day. A decision whose consequences you have to live with.

Along with healthy eating and anaerobic training, increasing cardio intensity will boost your metabolism and your insulin sensitivity.[341]

Interval training combines short high-intensity bursts of speed, with slow recovery phases, repeated during one exercise session. You can choose from the many cardio interval training routines available for free on the internet or you can ask a professional trainer you trust to recommend one for you.

Even though we're still talking about cardio exercises, interval training will earn you the prize of both fat burning aerobic effects and a higher metabolic anaerobic effect.[342] That is because during the short burst of extremely high intensity exercise, the muscles work without oxygen and accumulate lactic acid, entering into oxygen debt. And during the active relaxation recovery phases, the heart and the lungs work to cover this debt and break down the lactic acid muscle buildup. The recovery phase is very important, as this is the real fat burning phase.[343]

For instance, you can split the 30 minutes into 3 parts: 10 minutes warm up, 10 minutes interval training and 10 minutes cool down. This way the really hard part takes only 10 minutes. Start by gradually increasing your cardio exercise intensity from low to mid for the first 10 minutes warm up. Then go for the real fat loss! Each minute of the 10 minutes of actual interval training you must split in half. That is 30 seconds of cardio at a nearly all-out effort, followed by 30 seconds of low intensity cardio. Repeat this 10 times and you're done with the hard part. Then cool down by doing another 10 minutes of mid to low intensity cardio. This may sound simple, but some complete beginners might find it difficult to perform the 10 repetitions. So, start with 3 or 4 repetitions and then just cool down. Gradually increase the number of repetitions until you feel fit enough to perform the entire 10 minutes of this interval training. And remember that you don't just need to do it. For it to work, you have to do it right!

Another example is to do a 10 minutes warm up, followed by 5 combinations of 1 minute of the highest intensity cardio they can perform and 1 minute of low intensity cardio rest, and then cool down for 10 minutes. Also some people like to increase their cardio intensity in steps up to 3 or 4 minutes of their highest cardio level.

- So, how do you know which routine is best for you?

You will know the answer to this important question only after you've measured both the amount of time you can perform at your highest all-out effort intensity and the number of repetitions you were able to perform. Routines with stages of 3 or 4 minutes of extremely high intensity cardio might seem effective and the way to go for "the big boys." But my best bet is that most untrained people will not be able to sustain such a high level of physical effort for 2 or 3 minutes. You cannot choose a physical routine based on the fact that your trainer is able to do it. He is highly trained and his body can handle the effort of performing for 3 minutes at all-out effort. But, you are you; you are not him. And you will not end up looking like him (or her) if you over train. You will only end up quitting altogether.[344]

Educate yourself in everything you need to know about interval training before starting. Try different routines and choose the one that suits you. You can even create your own routine based on your own resistance to extremely high intensity exercise. Just don't forget to allow the warm up and cool down time. Warming up and cooling down might seem like a waste of time to some people, but they are of high importance in keeping you going in the long run.

The objective of the warm up is to raise total body temperature and muscle circulation, to prepare the body for the high intensity exercises. It prepares the cardiovascular, respiratory, nervous and muscular-skeletal systems by gradually increasing the intensity of the effort, so that they will be able to perform the higher intensity exercises. Also, warm up is of great importance when it comes to preventing injury.[345]

Stretching and cool down are just as important in reducing the risk of injury as the warm up. Gradually slowing down the intensity of your cardio exercises cools down your body and returns it to its normal state. The heart rate and respiration slow down gradually, and muscle soreness is prevented or at least delayed. When you skip cool down and suddenly stop your exercise, the lactic acid buildup remains in the muscles and causes swelling and pain. Cool down exercises ensure proper blood circulation to the muscles, enough to remove all or at least some of the lactic acid.[346] So, don't fool yourself by

skipping these important interval training phases.
Haste makes waste!

CHAPTER 24: HEALTHY FOODS

Healthy foods are nature-made foods.

-   What is the difference between man-made and nature-made foods?

Let me give you some examples. Nature made butter. Man made margarine and light butter. Nature made freshly squeezed orange juice. Man made bottled fortified or light orange juice. Nature made healthy wild salmon. Man made toxic farmed-like-fat-pigs salmon. Nature made full fat cheese. Man made light cheese and 0.1% fat "light" yoghurt. Nature made strawberries in June. Man-made strawberries all year round. Nature made taste-full tomatoes. Man made perfectly shaped tasteless tomatoes.

-   See the differences?

Fresh nature-made foods contain micronutrients and macronutrients. Man-made foods contain some micronutrients, some macronutrients and food additives, preservatives and even modified genes.[347]

The human body is designed to work on nature-made foods. Fueling your body with man-made foods implies accepting harm to your health, accepting the depositing of toxins in your body: that is, in the fat stores of your body.[348]

Eating a mainly natural, organic if possible, varied diet will ensure the optimum nutrient intake. All nutrients are needed for optimum health and many are missing from man-made foods, unless the food is "fortified" with the missing nutrient lost through food processing and storage. However, "fortifying" foods is not as healthy as it sounds.

For instance, while some calcium is naturally present in orange juice, we need to watch out that not too much is added to the "fortified orange juice", because calcium can form insoluble complexes with the pectin naturally contained by oranges. You might think:
- "Why should I watch out?
- Aren't doctors and scientists, the government or the food industry "watching out" for you?"

The brutally honest answer to this question is: "Not necessarily!"[349] Fortified foods with various micronutrients can be beneficiary only for people suffering from deficiencies, but they can also be a health hazard for people with normal micronutrient intakes.[350]

I know it sounds good, like buying "care" in a package. But it's just a promise. And this promise might not suit your own body's needs. Therefore, unless you have an objective blood analysis that proves you're deficient in some particular nutrient, just say "No" to fortified foods.[351]

Also, knowing what a food should contain in standard lab condition is not enough or even useful. I hear questions like "which contains more vitamin C, the green pepper or the orange juice?" all the time. People asking such questions either try to play smart, or have absolutely no idea, either about nutrition or about nutrients' bioavailability. The reality is that orange juice can contain zero vitamin C if you drink it a long time after squeezing.[352] And a green pepper can contain zero vitamin C, if you eat it in a salad chopped yesterday. You might think,

- "Who eats salad made with vegetables chopped a day or two before?"

Well... most salads sold in restaurants are chopped long before you buy them. And vitamin C oxidizes in about 15 minutes.[353]

- So what are you really eating?

We cannot just eat parsley, for optimum vitamin C intake. It must be freshly cut green parsley or the vitamin C is gone long before it reaches the mouth. And we cannot always choose fruits over sweets, just because the fruits are full of vitamins. If we really want cheese cake or ice cream and we eat apples or pineapple instead, in most cases we will end up eating both the fruits and the sweets. So, it's not just about combining food, macronutrients content, micronutrients content, or even just about hunger! A healthy varied diet must also provide the pleasure of eating, if we are to keep it up long-term.[354]

So, go ahead, slow down to the Fourth Gear and eat those commercially produced "empty" cookies if you really feel like eating them. Or drive in the Fifth Gear by choosing homemade cookies made with real eggs and full fat natural milk and sugar. Just don't rely on them to solve the sadness in your life. In spite of being a source of pleasure, food of any kind can only solve hunger. It is far safer and even more effective to rely on sports to solve unwanted feelings.[355]

It is scientifically proven that we need a certain intake of micronutrients for optimum health, but it is not proven that taking supplements containing any micronutrient will increase our state of health without a previous deficiency. Any "too much of a good thing" is a bad thing: supplements are not the exception to this rule![356] All the nutrients we need can be provided by a varied natural healthy diet, full of fruits, vegetables, raw nuts, seeds, grains, cold pressed extra virgin olive oil, wild fish, natural full-fat milk products, and organic eggs and meats coming from grass-fed animals.

You might like some food combinations, like cheese and tomatoes, or grilled meat and fresh salad. But eating the same foods every day is unhealthy, because no food out there will provide you with all the nutrients you need.[357] So, you must vary the foods you eat on a daily basis.

In the Fifth Gear you should eat only fresh, nature-made foods and vary them on daily basis to ensure optimum nutrient intake.

And by fresh, I don't mean uncooked. You can and really should cook some vegetables. And by all means, do cook your animal foods. By fresh I mean cooked or chopped now, just before eating. That is because the longer the time between cooking or chopping and the actual eating, the unhealthier that food becomes.[358]

- So, thinking about a fancy restaurant for dinner?

Think again! Most restaurants cook their food days before selling it to customers and keep it in refrigerators. Refrigerated food is not as healthy as fresh food. Therefore, unless you own the restaurant and really know that the food you're eating is fresh "for real," driving in the Fifth Gear means no eating at restaurants.

Also, you might think of some restaurants that cook the food in front of you, like in a "live cooking show". Really, open your eyes! Many foods used in a cooking show are precooked hours before the "show" and what you are actually witnessing is ... just a show.

If home cooking is not a part of your lifestyle, then just accept the Fourth Gear as your Top Gear.

Also, please don't fool yourself into thinking that "cooking" homemade pre-cooked refrigerated meals is healthy. It is not.[359] I'm not trying to confuse you even further. I'm trying to open your eyes. As I've said before, the Fifth Gear is very serious business. No more excuses.

As long as you keep introducing toxins into your body, you are fueling your fat tissue.

To be perfectly fit you must be perfectly healthy.

Driving in the Fifth Gear will get you to your dream body. But you must put in the effort by getting rid of the toxic foods that are holding you back and you must exercise every day.

CHAPTER 25 NUTRIENTS BIOAVAILABILITY

We take for granted that truth is contained in a lot of nutritional information. If a medical authority says it out loud, if it's written on some online dieting site, or if some celebrity doctor promotes it on his TV show, then it must be true.

- "I mean, these people are controlled by... the law people... or whatever people are put there to protect our health?"
- Right?

Trust me: no one is there to protect your health other than you. You are fully responsible for making educated choices about your health. I know it sounds like a big conspiracy, but it's really not. It's just free marketing. The food and weight loss industries are about profit, not about your health. And they have huge political influence, thus they are controlled to the minimum extent.

You are the one who is responsible for your health. *You* are the one who is responsible for your eating. *They* are just providing products to willing customers. Whether those products suit or don't suit your health needs is not their concern as long as they cause you to open your wallet. So, open your eyes instead and ask yourself:

- **"What am I eating?"**

- Does the food you are eating contain enough nutrients to ensure good health?
- And are those nutrients available for your body to use, just because you have eaten them?

A lot of factors like the quality of the soil, drought, herbicides used to control those plants, food processing, manner of cooking, food combinations in a meal, food preservatives the animals you eat were fed with or that are contained by their derived products, and even your health status all influence the bioavailability of nutrients.[360]

Let me give you a quick example of what I mean. I'm sure you have heard of Popeye, the scrawny sailor man who becomes super strong after eating spinach. Because spinach contains high levels of iron and calcium it is supposed to give you steel muscles! Well... even though a plate of spinach contains about the same amount of iron as a steak and about the same amount of calcium as a glass of milk, it also contains high levels of oxalic acid, which binds the iron,[361] and the calcium,[362] making them unusable to the human body.

- Now, you understand?

You just cannot know.

We are encouraged to audit our diets from food databases, to educate ourselves about which food contains what nutrients.

- Why do we need to know?

You would simply be wasting your time, as analyzing food is not even appropriate for macronutrients absorption and bioavailability, not to say completely inaccurate when it comes to micronutrients.[363] If you think that putting numbers on your foods is healthy, go for it, by all means.

- But what will those numbers mean for your health?

We do not absorb all the nutrients we take in, either from foods or from nutritional supplements.[364] We might even absorb none of the specific nutrients contained in some foods. Iron and calcium from spinach are healthy for the spinach itself, but have no value for humans.

Most vitamins are very well absorbed if the food is fresh, but vitamins' bioavailability decreases pretty fast after food processing of any sort takes place. And dietary minerals' bioavailability is even more complicated as it is influenced by so many factors.[365]

Let's say, for example, that you eat a big summer salad filled with all the vegetables you could find at the market and with some wild salmon, walnuts, parmesan and cold pressed extra virgin olive oil.

- Sounds healthy, right?

Well... let's take it one step at a time.

Humans do not absorb fiber, as you might know. You think you are doing wonders for your health by eating a big salad.

- But are you?

The fiber contained in the vegetables from your big salad will form a sifter on your intestinal wall, leaving less and less space through which the nutrients in your foods can be absorbed.[366] So every time you think a big salad is a good idea, really think! You can choose to enjoy the benefits of a denser intestinal sifter if you combine that big salad with fries or hamburgers or if you plan to enjoy some dessert. The fiber in your big salad will protect against the unhealthy fats or from the carbohydrate load.[367] But if you want to enjoy the benefits of the omega 3 from the wild salmon, walnuts and olive oil in your meal, then a big salad is not such a good idea anymore.

Use the fiber in foods as a protection whenever you want to eat something "unhealthy", but don't generalize and abuse them as "healthy food components". Too much fiber can harm you.[368]

So, no big salad unless you need it.

In addition, combining iron (from fish) and calcium (from the parmesan) is a very bad idea with regard to their bioavailability, because every time calcium and iron are taken together, the iron absorption can be decreased by up to 60%.[369] Calcium in both food and in dietary supplements has similar effects on decreasing iron absorption. Of course, it depends on the actual quantity of parmesan used in this salad. The point is: if you mix calcium (from sources like milk and cheese products, seeds, nuts or calcium supplements) and iron (from sources like meat, fish, or iron supplements) you will not absorb much of the iron. You might not care about it, you like your salad, it tastes good. But think about how many meat-cheese combinations we really eat! Too many! From the morning or lunch sandwich, to pizza, lasagna, and now even in salad; the meat iron in these dishes is not fully absorbed because of the calcium.

- Now, do you see the big picture?

Next in line is the omega 3 from the cold pressed extra virgin olive oil, from the walnuts and from the salmon. Omega 3 is like the definition of health.

- So this salad must be good for your health, right?

Yes. IF: the bottle of oil was opened less than a

207

couple of weeks ago and kept in a dark place.

No. IF: the salmon might have been overcooked or deep fried.

Overcooking or deep frying adulterates omega 3 fats. Overcooked salmon looks pink-white, starts flaking easily and looks dry. Smoked, salted and cured salmon loses about half of its original omega 3 content.[370] Raw fish is best for omega 3 levels, despite other possible health complications, such as microbe contamination and rancidity. If you cook the salmon yourself, pan-searing, baking and broiling are acceptable methods to maximize omega 3 bioavailability. Watch your salmon when cooking and make sure you stop cooking it before the flesh reaches full opacity, while it's still moist and red.

- So, are you beginning to understand the importance of home cooking?

Not only do you have greater control over the freshness of your food, but you can actually increase the bioavailability of the nutrients in your food, just by cooking your food the right way.

Nutrients bioavailability is so complex that you might not even want to deal with this concept.

Then, don't.

Just choose to **vary enough** the foods you eat on a daily basis, and be really careful about their freshness. You don't have to be a mechanic to be a fast driver.

You just have to be awake and aware.

CHAPTER 26: ANTIOXIDANTS

- Now, who thinks of cancer when they want to lose weight?

You should! We all should! Losing weight has become so present in everyone's lives that we have forgotten the fact that eating the wrong stuff might really hurt us. Some chase the weight loss fantasy to their death. Don't join the crowd!

Let us think a bit about free radicals, which are extremely important factors in the onset of cancer.[371] Free radicals are highly unstable and rapidly react with the nearest stable molecule, trying to steal the electron they need to reach a stable state. When the attacked molecule loses its electron, it becomes a free radical itself. Once the process is started, it can cascade, the domino effect damaging cellular compounds like DNA or cell membrane compounds, finally leading to the poor functioning or death of the cell or to extended life of a cell that should have died.

Some free radicals are produced during normal functions of the body, like hemoglobin breakdown, heat production, and muscle activity. And sometimes the body immune system's cells purposefully create free radicals to fight viruses, bacteria or against body cells like in type 1 diabetogenic process, which appears to be caused by immune destruction of the beta cells.[372]

In addition, environmental factors, such as exposure to pollution, radiation and tobacco, can increase the creation of free radicals.[373] Also, free radicals tend to accumulate inside body cells with age.[374] The damage done by free radicals is considered to be among the main causes of cancer, autoimmune disorders, cataract, rheumatoid arthritis, cardiovascular and neurodegenerative diseases.[375]

Since antioxidants equal "free radical damage control" they were chosen as the logical answer to an increased oxidative stress. The amazing idea that a daily pill could keep us disease-free and forever young has caught the eye of the pharmaceutical, food and weight loss industry. According to some estimates, around 40% of people take a daily antioxidant supplement.

It sounds almost too good to be true!

But before you go out and stock your pantry with antioxidant supplements, remember that more is not necessarily better. Some people might see antioxidant supplements as a harmless way of ensuring their health without the "fattening side effects" of foods. However, massive clinical trials are beginning to challenge this idea.

It is too good to be true!

Scientific evidence gathered over the past few years proves that at best, antioxidant supplements do little or nothing to enhance our health.[376] And at worst, they may harm our health. When speaking about the health benefits of using antioxidant supplements in order to prevent or treat cancer, many clinical trials have found that antioxidant supplements may <u>increased the risk</u> of:

1. developing some types of cancers;[377]
2. and of developing more aggressive forms of those cancers by protecting cancer cells from the destructive effects of cancer therapy. [378, 379]

In conclusion, if a supposedly protective substance acts as an antioxidant or has pro-oxidant activity, it is an area of current research.

The most worrisome of the antioxidants is vitamin E, because vitamin E supplements overuse may increase the risk of cardiovascular diseases, cancer and neurodegenerative disorders.[380] Moreover, some studies suggest that vitamin E supplementation may increase overall mortality,[381] and the risk of prostate cancer among healthy men.[382]

Although more research is needed in order to support or refute the findings of these studies, do not take vitamin E supplements if you suffer from any chronic disease; in fact, it's best avoid any supplementation unless prescribed by your physician.

Regarding fat loss, antioxidant supplements preclude the beneficial increase in muscles' insulin sensitivity that sport gives rise to. Researchers have scientifically proven that **exercise increases insulin sensitivity only in the absence of the antioxidant supplements**, both in previously untrained and trained individuals.[383] You might be a bit puzzled by the fact that 1 daily gram of vitamin C could negate the increase in insulin sensitivity gained through exercise. But this is objective science, not common sense trained subliminally by aggressive advertising. Because of their messing with sports' ability to decrease insulin resistance, antioxidants use might impede fat loss. Thus it is best to forget about any antioxidant supplements if you're trying to lose fat!

I never consider supplementation of any antioxidants, because the data about their possible interactions is questionable and unreliable.[384] For instance, smokers who took a beta carotene supplement in order to decrease the action of the extra free radicals resulting from smoking have shockingly discovered that the beta carotene itself increased the risk of lung cancer by almost 20%.[385]

A healthy lifestyle is the only way to go when it comes to controlling the production of free radicals. Antioxidants naturally found in fruits and vegetables have the potential to improve and maintain proper health. The easiest way to get enough antioxidants is to eat plenty of fresh vegetal food.

So be safe and eat your antioxidants.

Don't "take" them!

CHAPTER 27: DIETARY SUPPLEMENTS

Many people out there rely on supplements when they go on weird diets.

-   But can we really know if taking a vitamin or mineral supplement will be enough to ensure our health during a crazy diet?

Most individuals taking vitamin and mineral supplements expect to be less tired without resting accordingly, to feel better without eating properly, to improve their appearance without physical activity and proper eating, to perform better without considering the natural limits of their body, or to prevent diseases without making lifestyle changes.

There is so much questionable information out there and we are so encouraged to take vitamin and mineral supplements that most of us don't really know what to do when it comes to these supplements. About half of the population should take a daily supplement of some sort, in some scientists' opinion. But despite the beliefs of these "scientists" and the pharmaceutical industry shareholders, relatively few supplements are really vital for proper health and even fewer supplements are as effective as they promise to be.[386]

However, due to intensive marketing, dietary supplements are becoming more and more popular.

People get attracted by the health claims of the manufacturers and, sometimes, they substitute a healthy diet for these supplements. But taking vitamin and mineral supplements without professional advice may lead to health problems, due to the toxicity of high doses of micronutrients or due to interactions between micronutrients.[387] So, to start with, avoid any vitamin or mineral supplement unless prescribed by a health care provider.

To explain the dangers of supplements, I'll use calcium as an example.

Because the need for calcium goes up from 1000 mg per day in pre-menopausal women to 1200 mg per day for post-menopausal women, post-menopausal women are encouraged to take calcium and vitamin D supplements. However, studies have linked calcium and vitamin D supplements with increased heart attack risk.[388] Some epidemiological studies also indicate that high calcium intake is associated with increased risk of prostate cancer,[389] but more research is needed in order to be able to make a medically accurate recommendation regarding this issue.

- Do you start to see the big picture?

Dietary supplements are not as harmless and as health protective as they are promoted to be! People with chronic diseases or lowered immunity should never take a vitamin or mineral supplement, unless supervised by their doctor. The supplements might interact with medication and can even be detrimental to breast cancer patients.[390] In order to increase immunity you must eat right, rest well, engage in regular physical exercises and be as happy as you can be every moment of our lives.

As far as taking vitamin C to prevent colds,[391] or other vitamins and minerals to prevent chronic diseases,[392] there is not enough evidence to support this theory. Also, vitamin C is water soluble, which means that if you take one pill containing a full daily vitamin C requirement, you will use the quantity you need at the moment and excrete all the rest through urine. Maybe taking vitamin C could shorten the duration of a cold by a day or two, but also intakes larger than 2000 mg can cause nasty symptoms like diarrhea.[393] So take your pick!

Supplements need to be considered in the same light as medicinal products and should undergo strict evaluation before marketing. In Europe, supplements must have been demonstrated to be safe, both in dosages and in purity, but they can bear health claims without supporting scientific evidence.[394]

But in US dietary supplements do not need to be pre-tested before they can enter the market.[395] To the dismay of many scientists, US dietary supplements are legally defined as "a product that is intended to supplement the diet and contains any of the following dietary ingredients: a vitamin, a mineral, an herb or other botanical (excluding tobacco), an amino acid, a concentrate, metabolite, constituent, extract, or combination of any of the above, a substance historically used by humans to supplement the diet. It must also conform to the following criteria: "intended for ingestion in pill, capsule, tablet, powder or liquid form, not represented for use as a conventional food or as the sole item of a meal or diet, labeled as a <dietary supplement>." That's it! This quoted legal definition of US supplements contains nothing about the legality of health claims, nothing about supplement labeling regulations and nothing about the lack of information on side effects! Their legal definition is not about their safety or about their effectiveness in enhancing health, but about their content!

People assume that supplements don't have side effects, because such side effects are not written on their label. But unlike the pharmaceutical industry, manufacturers of dietary supplements **are not required by the law** to prove the bioavailability of their products, the health promoting effectiveness, or the absence of side effects.

And please keep in mind that this chapter is not a statement against dietary supplements manufacturers in favor of the Big Pharma companies. This is not what I mean at all. Also do not forget that most dietary supplements are produced and marketed by the same Big Pharma companies that also control the pharmaceutical market. What I need you to understand is that the laws regulating dietary supplements are elusive, making these products easier to promote and sell by their manufacturers.

To sum it all up, always remember that there is no substitute for healthy eating. Supplements should only complement a healthy diet when objectively needed, not replace it.

CHAPTER 28: WEIGHT LOSS MEDICATION

- Can weight loss medication cure obesity?
- And is weight loss medication generating fat loss or weight loss?

You might not care about the answers to these questions. Many people don't care about these answers. So many people out there just take weight loss pills and never read the medical information leaflets provided with them. They know deep down that the side effects can be severe.[396] Some even know or will soon find out that they'll have to wear diapers while taking such medication.[397] But some are so desperate that they don't care. They want to lose weight no matter what! And the other weight loss pill users are just looking for an easy solution to their weight gain problem.

- Is there a cozy way out of the weight gain problem?

If asked, any marketing expert will tell you that there are no problems, only challenges. And even though you might consider obesity a problem, the pharmaceutical industry is here to save the day. It has and continues to develop new medication to overcome any challenge weight gain could pose. From medication that inhibits intestinal absorption of fats that at the same time saves you from fat's "extra calories" and makes you shit your pants, to medication that both increases adipocytes lipolysis and the risk of stroke,[398] they've thought up any possible ways to help you overcome obesity challenges. But this is what marketing is. This is not human physiology. This is marketing departments searching for loopholes in human physiology.

This is about selling stuff, not about you. Yes you, the fat people, are important. You get to see the marketing show and have the marketing executives down at your feet offering to solve your challenges for you.

- Are you willing to pay for others to solve your weight gain challenges for you?

Most people would be. Harry Potter was a huge success, because people believe in magic.

- Do you buy that popping some pills into your system will solve your weight problem?

Of course you do. Literally.

You even buy ketone strips to prove... what?

Because if you've really been there with me as I've taught you how to drive in the Second Gear, then you must have understood that ketosis only happens when the metabolism of fatty acids is incomplete due to the oxaloacetate shortage (please read that Gear again if you need to remember this). Ketosis equals incomplete fatty acids metabolization and storage within the muscle cell, further aggravating muscle insulin resistance. But you didn't know that.

And the weight loss industry people know that you didn't. See, they are smart. And they've done their homework on knowing their target audience really well. For example, Asia has the potential to hugely increase the weight loss industry's profits.[399] But despite the fact that Asians are willingly embracing the "western" lifestyle, thus becoming fatter, they are also more prone to healthy eating. So, the weight loss marketing directions for Asians are focused on "healthy diet plans", on vitamin and mineral supplements, and weight loss pills.

It's all about money.

Your money.

And they really want is your money.

-    Is their behavior unethical?

Maybe. You are a willing buyer. They're selling solutions. It's your job to decide if their solutions suit your personal needs. No one is responsible, but you, for your buying decisions.

However, medication should be used only to treat real diseases and only under medical supervision. Being overweight or obese is a causal factor for many life-threatening diseases. But it is induced by an unhealthy lifestyle and it should be treated through improved lifestyle.

Also, the laws regulating weight loss medication should call for mandatory physician prescription,[400] since these over-the-counter weight loss drugs have severe side effects.[401] But nowadays the weight loss industry's shareholders are stronger than ever. They make the laws and they make them with the purpose of increasing profit, not with the purpose of ending the obesity epidemic.

- **How would the end of the obesity epidemic serve them?**

The ones holding power dictate what's right and what's wrong, according to their profit margins. You follow. This is what the free market is all about.

Or should I say jungle...

Fifth Gear Recap:

Small-step goal no. 1:_**Eat only when and only for as long as you are biologically hungry.**

Never eat food you dislike *

Sleep enough *

Don't use any electrical weight loss procedure *

Small-step goal no. 3:_**Eat both vegetal and animal foods when hungry.**

Small-step goal no. 4: **Hydrate yourself with at least 1 liter of water every day.**

Limit yourself to one coffee and one alcoholic drink/ a day *

Don't drink soft drinks or weight loss teas *

After successfully achieving the goal no. 4 on a daily basis, you can either attempt to also achieve small-step goals no. 5 and 6, or you can settle with the Fourth Gear as your top one and move straight to the Maintenance stage. As with everything about fat loss, this is a personal choice!

Small-step goal no. 5: **Do 30 minutes interval training cardio/ 30 minutes anaerobic exercises every day.**

Small-step goal no. 6: **Eat only fresh & diversified nature-made foods.**

Don't eat precooked food at restaurants or at home *

Don't take antioxidants, supplements or weight loss pills *

* These are not mandatory goals, but they might sabotage your fat loss unless taken into consideration.

CHAPTER 29: CAN CHILDREN DRIVE?

Nowadays, children seem to be worrying about their weight and body image at an ever younger age. That is why preventing and treating obesity in children starts with what their parents do. That is with what the parents **do**, not with what the parents **say**.

-   **Should fat children diet?**

I analyze this topic in great depth in my book on children nutrition "Nutrition Guide for Mums", but let's talk a bit about what parents do to bring about the onset of childhood obesity.

Many parents set fixed eating schedules for their babies.

-   Are these fixed meal times in the best interest of the children or in the parents' best interest?
-   What has the child to gain from a fixed meal

time schedule?

Ask yourself these questions, because if you think about it, a fixed eating schedule is the foundation for the separation of hunger and eating.[402] These parents are teaching their children from day one that eating is not about hunger. These children have to eat when their parents arbitrarily decide, not when they feel hungry. Children are born with the perfect hunger-eating-satiation system, but many are not allowed to use it, because their parents know better. However, eating is not controlled in the conscious part of the human brain.

- So, how can these parents know better?
- And what do they know better?

They are teaching their children that decisions about how much food they eat should be based on what it says in a book, or what is advised by the doctors, not about the quantity children feel is enough. Such parents are treating their children as unreliable when it comes to eating behavior.

- In what way are these parents reliable?

They don't allow children to follow their hunger or they are worried when the children aren't eating "enough."

- Enough for whom?

I know that everybody raises their children as they wish, but still! If left on their own, children would not die of hunger with healthy food available.

The inborn eating behavior of our children is the most powerful tool we can use to prevent childhood obesity. But it is very hard to accept for lifelong dieter parents, parents who usually end up with the highest percentage of overweight or obese children.[403] So, don't create meal schedules for your children. I know it can be tiring and scary to let go of controlling your child's eating. But look around you! We all live in a society fatter than ever, with children fatter than ever.

Some parents may argue that their children would eat only sweets if they could. Sometimes this can be true, but we can only educate our children about healthy foods through personal example and through encouragement. After that, it is just a matter of trust in the human biology. And biology is there, deep in our hypothalamus, from birth. Allowing your children to use their own internal hunger-eating-satiation cues is a tool they'll benefit from all their life! Therefore, it is of huge importance to try your best to respect children's hunger despite your daily to-do list.[404]

Of course, some children can play so much that they forget about hunger, then become too hungry and overeat. But although this can happen sometimes, always reinforce eating only when and only for as long hunger is in the picture. So invite them to eat while still playing, ask them if they are hungry and accept their answers. Emphasize hunger instead of obedience!

Also, please try your best to dismiss eating as a sign of courtesy. When they're not hungry, accept their participation in family dinners without eating. Teach your children that family dinners should be about sharing quality time, not about mandatory eating. And do all this because the main root cause of obesity is that eating is almost never about hunger. Eating the most tasteful healthy food available when hunger does exist is one of the most important obesity preventive skills we can teach our children.

Mothers who are overly concerned about their children's weight and physical attractiveness may put them at increased risk of developing obesity or eating disorders.[405] Many girls with eating disorders have a parent, brothers or friends who are overly critical of their weight.[406] Also, obese parents tend to handle food issues and weight concerns differently than parents who never diet.[407] They impose patterns that include fixed, rigid feeding schedules and use food for non-nutritive purposes like punishment or reward. Moreover, many parents and grandparents comfort or bribe children with food. This is one of the most powerful factors that lead to hunger/eating separation. Later in life these children will use food to pamper their "wounds", causing many to increase the number of overweight or obese people.[408]

So: never use food as a reward, punishment or comfort for unwanted feelings or situations.

Children of parents with dieting history have a higher risk of becoming obese than those whose parents have no food or weight issues.[409] That is because children learn attitudes about eating and self value through observation, attitudes that are often copied. When mom rests her self-worth on her appearance and is dissatisfied with her body and diets frequently, her children will learn to do the same.

Families that include one or more dieters tend to be overprotective, rigid and unsuccessful at resolving conflicts. Children of such families are taught not to discuss fears, doubts, imperfections or failures. Instead of trying to solve the roots of their problems, they rely on manipulating their weight and food intake to express their feelings and difficulties.[410] Social and cultural expectations can also be cruel and unrelenting towards thinness.

But dieting triggers obesity.[411]

Thus children should never diet. Ever.

Besides, diets don't work in the long run,[412] and whatever weight is lost, it will never be enough. Teaching children "tools" to help them build strong selves and teaching them to cope with their feelings, educating them about healthy eating and encouraging them to engage in fun physical activities are the key factors that prevent obesity and eating disorders.

Children's obesity is preventable, but all the hard work starts with the parents. Anything you do as a parent speaks louder than anything you say. A healthy role model is a child's best protection against many of life's problems, including obesity. So make the effort and associate your own healthy eating with a healthy beautiful body. Stick to a nutritious eating and promote fun sport activities as a way of controlling your weight. Make time for family meals and serve healthy natural tasty foods, and don't forget deserts! Banning certain foods, for any reason, will just make your children binge on them.[413] Any food can be eaten in moderation. Also, pay attention to the fact that watching food as a source of calories and fat grams can become obsessive easily. Food brings us the pleasure of eating it, not just energy or vitamins.

Never criticize your own body in your children's presence. Learn to love your own body and make the effort it needs for you to like it. Whenever a parent criticizes their body, the child becomes overly concerned about his own body. Remember kids follow their parent's lead, so behavior is passed down to a child, whether it seems harmless or not. Never joke about a child's body, or anyone's for that matter. Praise your children's positive qualities and their accomplishments, not how they look. We are not put on this planet to send all our time beautifying ourselves. We have talents, abilities, hopes, dreams, values and goals. Physical appearance is just the outer shell. Allowing anyone to tease your children about their appearance can produce powerful negative consequences and low self-esteem.[414] Many parents, especially fathers or lifelong dieter mothers think that if they are the ones critical of their child's body, it will somehow make the child stronger and the child will be more able to deal with everyday cruel life.[415]

Your child won't become stronger and more prepared "for what is out there" if you harm him yourself.

All parents should offer unconditional love and support; they should not harm children in order for them to become accustomed to a tough life. Children are not miniature adults! They are emotionally vulnerable persons that must be taught how to healthily cope with their feelings, so that they don't rely on their body weight as a barometer for their self-worth as humans. Learning how to express "good" and "bad" feelings, and that it is important to express them, is key to preventing juvenile obesity.

By listening to your children and sharing their emotions, you can make them less likely to use food or starvation as a way of expressing anger, frustration, happiness, sadness, or as a way of dealing with boredom. If your children have troubles letting out some of their feelings, encourage them to communicate those feelings in a non-verbal way, through writing, painting, or even running or dancing. Also, encourage your children to form quality trusting relationships with other adults, to whom they can go if they have an issue that they would consider unsuitable for a parent's ear.

And do talk to your children about the "perfect" images promoted through media and explain to them that some of the perceived images are false. Nowadays pictures can be easily modified according to the commercial message intended to be perceived. Also, many of the models and actresses achieve a thin body only through extreme diets, drugs and plastic surgery, not through healthy eating and sports. But these famous people make a living out of their looks, thus they are pressured to force their bodies thin through whatever means necessary. Point out to your children that the advertiser's target population is made up of people with body image insecurities and that the slimming products are not meant to help them achieve happiness, but temporary thinness.

The only reason behind marketing slimness is profit. And the product that increases self-esteem has not been invented yet.

CHAPTER 30: FEAR FACTOR

An old German proverb goes: "Fear makes the wolf bigger than he is." The oldest and strongest emotion is fear, a vital response to physical or emotional danger. But the change that healthy eating and sports can bring is far from putting you into danger. If you need to lose fat, but the fear of stepping outside the dieting world is holding you back, ask yourself these questions:

- What is the best outcome that can happen?
- What is the worst outcome that can happen?
- And can you lose fat and keep it off without changing your lifestyle?

I think it's very important to ask yourself all these questions before starting any diet.

I will start by addressing the last question, because so many fat people out there expect to become thin with as little change as possible. The main question in such people's minds is:

- "How much can I eat and still lose weight?" and not:
- "How can I eat less?"

But if you are fat, you must get out of your current comfort zone and create a new one. There is no shortcut to thinness! You must assume that you are responsible for the quality of your life. You cannot eat mindlessly, be sedentary and lose fat, no matter what crazy miracle diet you follow. You cannot just take some pills, drink some weight loss laxative teas and eat low-fat foods to become thin. You cannot just count calories, or points or fat grams or whatever, and lose fat.

There is no cozy way out of obesity.

Fat loss and weight maintenance require personal effort. These are long term processes not events, they don't just happen! And when the going gets rough, you will want to give up.

Don't.

Most people just assume the outcome of any diet as weight loss, implies fat loss. Thus, they base their actions on wishful thinking and expect the best results they've heard of. They're putting their fate into the hands of diet gurus or anyone else they think might have a clue about weight loss. Some make all the effort they can sustain; some start at a fast pace then just quit; others live continuously on and off a diet. Surely more than half of the fat people out there are deeply unhappy with their bodies and with the solutions scientists are offering to the obesity problem[416]. Yet only a tiny fraction is complaining about the inefficiency of diets or scientists' inability to "fix" this worldwide health problem.

-   Why do people withhold their complaints?

Their shame and guilt express their fear of stepping outside the herd. Many fat people feel embarrassed and humiliated by the lack of effective solutions to their weight problem offered by the weight loss industry, and yet they continue to pay their share.

-   Shouldn't the weight loss industry pay back?

Moreover, many fat people feel blamed by the medical system when it comes to weight loss[417]. They are required to swallow contradictory guidelines from medical authorities more and more confused and overwhelmed by the obesity epidemic. They've put their trust in science and have stopped trusting their own bodies[418]. They've put their trust in the society and have stopped trusting what feels right for them. And besides inefficiency, society harms them even more by saying they lack willpower.

-   How long are you going to stand there and take this?

Some of you might be thinking that facing fear every day sounds like an awful way to live. But the only thing you have to fear is fear itself. Courage is not the lack of fear but the ability to face it. It is hard! I agree. But fear is not a reason for passivity, it is only an excuse. And fear doesn't exist anywhere except in your mind. It is like a wild animal. It is a coward, but it will attack if it sees you are afraid of it. But if you hold your ground, it will disappear.

Fat people put their lives on hold, because they are afraid to make a lifestyle change. But success carries responsibility with it. You are responsible for achieving it, you have no one to blame, but yourself.

It is easier to postpone real fat loss efforts and dream your life away on the "when I'm thin, I will..." mentality. Somebody should have told you at birth that you are dying with every passing second. Then, maybe, you would have lived every minute of your life.

Too many fat people are fat because they are living in fear. The other side of fear is freedom.

THE END?

When I first imagined this book, I wanted to write something spectacular as a Grand Finale. But now, now that I have actually succeeded in writing it, I feel I've said enough. Now it is your turn!

The end is up to you.

However, as I mentioned at the beginning of this book, please keep in mind that the weight loss industry shareholders expect to transform almost half of us into overweight or obese slaves by 2020[419]. What I'm telling you is that you actually have to decide now in which half of the population you'll be then! You can do the hard work and enjoy the freedom of driving a slim fit body or you can just take the cozy fatty subway like everyone else. This is your decision to take.

And if achieving the small-step goals in this book seems like more work and commitment than you can handle, don't worry, I understand!

It is not your fault that you're going to be late for...

It is not you driving your body fat or slim.

It is not you who's responsible.

But it will always be you who has to live with or die by the consequences of your silent decisions. It will always be your life on hold.

Passivity is a choice. I accept your choice.

- Do you?

Look at you, and decide.

HOW TO APPLY THE METHOD:

Master each Small-step Goal before even considering the next one. Jumping straight to the Fifth Gear will either give you the wrong idea or make you quit before you can reap any rewards. So, take it as slow as you did when you learned how to drive a car.

Small-step Goal no. 1: **Eat only when and only for as long as you are biologically hungry.**

Never eat food that you dislike *

Sleep enough *

Although consciously braking is the basis of self-control, when it comes to building the habit of only eating when hungry, it is effective to consider it achieved only after 1 full week without any braking.

This goal should be achieved and practiced on a daily basis for at least 1 week before starting to learn how to drive in the Second Gear!

Small-step goal no. 2: **Do 30 minutes of cardio/anaerobic exercises every other day.**

Don't use any electrical weight loss procedure *

Please do not start to drive in the Third Gear before mastering and practicing the first two goals on a daily basis, for at least 1 full week!

Small-step goal no. 3: **Eat both vegetal and animal foods when hungry.**

After successfully achieving goal no. 3 on a daily basis for more than 1 week, you end the Preparation stage of your changing progress. Please do not start to work on the Fourth Gear until mastering and practicing the first 3 ones for at least 1 week!

Small step goal no. 4: **Hydrate yourself with at least 1 liter of water every day.**

Limit yourself to one coffee and one alcoholic drink/ day *

Don't drink soft drinks or weight loss teas *

After successfully achieving the goal no. 4 on a daily basis, you can either attempt to also achieve small-step goals no. 5 and 6, or you can settle with the Fourth Gear as your top one and move straight to the Maintenance stage. As with everything about fat loss, this is a personal choice!

Small-step goal no. 5: **Do 30 minutes interval training cardio/ 30 minutes anaerobic exercises every day.**

Small-step goal no. 6: **Eat only fresh & diversified nature-made foods.**

Don't eat precooked food at restaurants or at home *

Don't take antioxidants, supplements or weight loss pills *

After a period of six months to a year of driving mainly in the 4th and 5th Gears without relapses, move on to improve other areas in your life.

* These are not mandatory goals, but they might sabotage your fat loss unless taken into consideration.

ABOUT THE AUTHOR

Diana Artene is a licensed physical therapist since 2003. After she graduated Medical University she extended her medical knowledge in sport nutrition, nutrition for weight loss and children nutrition as she became a nutritionist.

She advocates a healthy lifestyle in which all foods can be eaten and no long workouts are necessary to be fit and slim as long as we are fully informed.

She's also the author of:

Nutrition Guide for Mums: Healthy eating tips for you and your children

NOTE FROM AUTHOR

Thank you for purchasing and reading this book. I am positive it will help you with your fat loss and health goals!

Your opinion is very important to me. Kindly consider leaving an honest review on Amazon, or on other book-related sites, such as Goodreads or LibraryThing.

Also, if you have any questions or need some help to apply the 5 Gears Diet, please send me an email using the contact form at www.artenediana.com.

I'll be happy to help you!

BIBLIOGRAPHY

1: World Health Organization, Obesity and Overweight Fact sheet N°311 (updated March 2013): http://www.who.int/mediacentre/factsheets/fs311/en/

2: Finucane MM, Stevens GA, Cowan MJ, et al. National, regional, and global trends in body-mass index since 1980: systematic analysis of health examination surveys and epidemiological studies with 960 country-years and 9.1 million participants. *Lancet.* 2011;377:557-67. http://www.hsph.harvard.edu/obesity-prevention-source/obesity-trends/obesity-rates-worldwide/

3: Kelly T, Yang W, Chen CS, Reynolds K, He J. Global burden of obesity in 2005 and projections to 2030.*Int J Obes (Lond).* 2008;32:1431-7.

4: Weight Management Market by Services, Supplements, Diet, Equipment and Devices: Global Analysis And Forecast (2007 - 2015) http://www.businesswire.com/news/home/20120201006303/en/Global-Weight-Management-Market-Analysis-Forecast-MarketPublishers.com

5: WHITING, David R., et al. IDF diabetes atlas: global estimates of the prevalence of diabetes for 2011 and 2030. *Diabetes research and clinical practice*, 2011, 94.3: 311-321.

6: FINKELSTEIN, Eric A., et al. Obesity and severe obesity forecasts through 2030. *American journal of preventive medicine*, 2012, 42.6: 563-570.

7: HANKEY, C. R., et al. Eating habits, beliefs, attitudes and knowledge among health professionals regarding the links between obesity, nutrition and health. *Public health nutrition*, 2004, 7.02: 337-343.

8: SAPER, Clifford B.; CHOU, Thomas C.; ELMQUIST, Joel K. The need to feed: homeostatic and hedonic control of eating. *Neuron*, 2002, 36.2: 199-211.

9: STUNKARD, Albert. Obesity and the denial of hunger. *Psychosomatic Medicine*, 1959, 21.4: 281-289.

10: Ania M. Jastreboff, Rajita Sinha, Cheryl Lacadie, Dana M. Small, Robert S. Sherwin, and Marc N. Potenza. Neural Correlates of Stress- and Food Cue–Induced Food Craving in Obesity: Association with insulin levels Diabetes Care February 2013 36:394-402; published ahead of print. October 15, 2012, doi:10.2337/dc12-1112

11: LEVY, Alan S.; HEATON, Alan W. Weight control practices of US adults trying to lose weight. *Annals of Internal Medicine*, 1993, 119.7_Part_2: 661-666.

12: HEBERT, James R., et al. Scientific Decision Making, Policy Decisions, and the Obesity Pandemic. In: *Mayo Clinic Proceedings*. Elsevier, 2013. p. 593-604.

13: THOMPSON, Donald B.; MCDONALD, Bryan. What Food is "Good" for You? Toward a Pragmatic Consideration of Multiple Values Domains. *Journal of Agricultural and Environmental Ethics*, 2013, 26.1: 137-163.

14: GUTHRIE, Helen A.; SCHEER, James C. Nutritional adequacy of self-selected diets that satisfy the four food groups guide. *Journal of Nutrition Education*, 1981, 13.2: 46-49.

15: DIXON, Lori Beth; CRONIN, Frances J.; KREBS-SMITH, Susan M. Let the pyramid guide your food choices: capturing the total diet concept. *The Journal of nutrition*, 2001, 131.2: 461S-472S.

16: DE WITT HUBERTS, Jessie C.; EVERS, Catharine; DE

RIDDER, Denise TD. Double trouble: restrained eaters do not eat less and feel worse. *Psychology & health*, 2013, 28.6: 686-700.

17: POLIVY, Janet; HERMAN, C. Peter. Dieting and binging: a causal analysis.*American Psychologist*, 1985, 40.2: 193.

18: WESTENHOEFER, Joachim, et al. Cognitive control of eating behavior and the disinhibition effect. *Appetite*, 1994, 23.1: 27-41.

19: LENDERS, Carine, et al. A Novel Nutrition Medicine Education Model: the Boston University Experience. *Advances in Nutrition: An International Review Journal*, 2013, 4.1: 1-7.

20: BLOCK, Jason P.; DESALVO, Karen B.; FISHER, William P. Are physicians equipped to address the obesity epidemic? knowledge and attitudes of internal medicine residents☆. *Preventive medicine*, 2003, 36.6: 669-675.

21: EISENBERG, David M., et al. Enhancing Medical Education to Address Obesity:"See One. Taste One. Cook One. Teach One.". *JAMA internal medicine*, 2013, 1-3.

22: SWIFT, J. A.; SHEARD, C.; RUTHERFORD, M. Trainee health care professionals' knowledge of the health risks associated with obesity. *Journal of Human Nutrition and Dietetics*, 2007, 20.6: 599-604.

23: FAROOQUI, Akhlaq A. Lifestyle as a Risk Factor for Metabolic Syndrome and Neurological Disorders. In: *Metabolic Syndrome*. Springer New York, 2013. p. 1-34.

24: DAVISON, K. K.; MARKEY, C. N.; BIRCH, L. L. Etiology of body dissatisfaction and weight concerns among 5-year-old girls. *Appetite*, 2000, 35.2: 143-151.

25: ADAMS, Peter J., et al. Body dissatisfaction, eating disorders, and depression: A developmental perspective. *Journal of Child and Family Studies*, 1993, 2.1: 37-46.

26: SCHWARTZ, Marlene B.; BROWNELL, Kelly D. Obesity and body image. *Body image*, 2004, 1.1: 43-56.

27: WILSON, G. Terence. Acceptance and change in the treatment of eating disorders and obesity. *Behavior Therapy*, 1996, 27.3: 417-439.

28: YANG, Qing. Gain weight by "going diet?" Artificial sweeteners and the neurobiology of sugar cravings: Neuroscience 2010. *The Yale journal of biology and medicine*, 2010, 83.2: 101.

29: SHROFF, Hemal, et al. Features associated with excessive exercise in women with eating disorders. *international Journal of Eating disorders*, 2006, 39.6: 454-461.

30: POLIVY, Janet; HERMAN, C. Peter. Diagnosis and treatment of normal eating. *Journal of consulting and clinical psychology*, 1987, 55.5: 635.

31: CANETTI, Laura; BACHAR, Eytan; BERRY, Elliot M. Food and emotion. *Behavioural processes*, 2002, 60.2: 157-164.

32: NESTLE, Marion. The ironic politics of obesity. *Science*, 2003, 299.5608: 781-781.

33: WARDLE, Jane; BEALES, Sally. Control and loss of control over eating: An experimental investigation. *Journal of Abnormal Psychology*, 1988, 97.1: 35.

34: OCHNER, Christopher N., et al. Biological Mechanisms that Promote Weight Regain Following Weight Loss in Obese Humans. *Physiology & behavior*, 2013.

35: SAGAYAMA, Hiroyuki, et al. Effects of rapid weight loss and regain on body composition and energy expenditure. *Applied Physiology, Nutrition, and Metabolism*, 2013, ja.

36: ELLIOT, Diane L., et al. Sustained depression of the resting metabolic rate after massive weight loss. *The American journal of clinical nutrition*, 1989, 49.1: 93-96.

37: MACLEAN, Paul S., et al. Biology's response to dieting: the impetus for weight regain. *American Journal of Physiology-Regulatory, Integrative and Comparative Physiology*, 2011, 301.3: R581-R600.

38: FEDOROFF, Ingrid; POLIVY, Janet; PETER HERMAN, C. The

specificity of restrained versus unrestrained eaters' responses to food cues: general desire to eat, or craving for the cued food?. *Appetite*, 2003, 41.1: 7-13.

39: MANN, Traci, et al. Medicare's search for effective obesity treatments: diets are not the answer. *American Psychologist*, 2007, 62.3: 220.

40: TANOFSKY-KRAFF, Marian; YANOVSKI, Susan Z. Eating Disorder or Disordered Eating? Non-normative Eating Patterns in Obese Individuals. *Obesity research*, 2004, 12.9: 1361-1366.

41: BUNTON, Robin, et al. The 'stages of change' model in health promotion: science and ideology. *Critical Public Health*, 2000, 10.1: 55-70.

42: KAYMAN, Susan; BRUVOLD, William; STERN, Judith S. Maintenance and relapse after weight loss in women: behavioral aspects. *The American journal of clinical nutrition*, 1990, 52.5: 800-807.

43: ELFHAG, K.; RÖSSNER, S. Who succeeds in maintaining weight loss? A conceptual review of factors associated with weight loss maintenance and weight regain. *Obesity reviews*, 2005, 6.1: 67-85.

44: CIAMPOLINI, Mario, et al. Hunger can be taught: Hunger Recognition regulates eating and improves energy balance. *International Journal of General Medicine*, 2013, 6: 465-478.

45: REINA, Samantha A., et al. Sociocultural pressures and adolescent eating in the absence of hunger. *Body image*, 2013.

46: SAINSBURY, A.; ZHANG, L. Role of the arcuate nucleus of the hypothalamus in regulation of body weight during energy deficit. *Molecular and cellular endocrinology*, 2010, 316.2: 109-119.

47: GOLAN, Moria; CROW, Scott. Parents are key players in the prevention and treatment of weight-related problems. *Nutrition reviews*, 2004, 62.1: 39-50.

48: HEATHERTON, Todd F.; POLIVY, Janet; HERMAN, C. Peter. Restraint and internal responsiveness: Effects of placebo manipulations of hunger state on eating. *Journal of Abnormal Psychology*, 1989, 98.1: 89.

49: KOOPMAN, Karin E., et al. Diet-induced changes in the Lean Brain: Hypercaloric High-Fat-High-Sugar Snacking decreases Serotonin Transporters the human hypothalamic region. *Molecular Metabolism*, 2013.

50: APPELHANS, Bradley M. Neurobehavioral Inhibition of Reward-driven Feeding: Implications for Dieting and Obesity. *Obesity*, 2009, 17.4: 640-647.

51: BERRIDGE, Kent C. Modulation of taste affect by hunger, caloric satiety, and sensory-specific satiety in the rat. *Appetite*, 1991, 16.2: 103-120.

52: TYLKA, Tracy L. Development and psychometric evaluation of a measure of intuitive eating. *Journal of Counseling Psychology*, 2006, 53.2: 226.

53: DAVIS, Caroline. From Passive Overeating to "Food Addiction": A Spectrum of Compulsion and Severity. *ISRN Obesity*, 2013, 2013.

54: OUTLAND, Lauren; RUST, Frank. Why Disrupt Homeostasis? Reasons Given for Not Eating When Hungry and Not Stopping When Full. *Holistic Nursing Practice*, 2013, 27.4: 239-245.

55:http://www.nobelprize.org/educational/medicine/pavlov/readmore.html

56: SWITHERS, Susan E. Artificial sweeteners produce the counterintuitive effect of inducing metabolic derangements. *Trends in Endocrinology & Metabolism*, 2013.

57: University of California, Berkeley: The Digestive System: http://mcb.berkeley.edu/courses/mcb32/Miller%20notes-%20digestive%20system%20

58: Gonnissen HKJ, Mazuy C, Rutters F, Martens EAP, Adam TC, et al. (2013) Sleep Architecture When Sleeping at an Unusual Circadian Time and Associations with Insulin Sensitivity. PLoS ONE 8(8): e72877. doi:10.1371/journal.pone.0072877

59: WOLK, Robert, et al. Sleep and cardiovascular disease. *Current problems in cardiology*, 2005, 30.12: 625-662.

60: KIM, Ji Young; HAN, Sang-Hwan; YANG, Bong-Min. Implication of high-body-fat percentage on cardiometabolic risk in middle-aged, healthy, normal-weight adults. *Obesity*, 2013.

61: BODEN, Guenther. Free fatty acids (FFA), a link between obesity and insulin resistance. *Front Biosci*, 1998, 3: d169-d175.

62: KOFFLER, Michael; KISCH, Eldad S. Starvation diet and very-low-calorie diets may induce insulin resistance and overt diabetes mellitus. *Journal of Diabetes and its Complications*, 1996, 10.2: 109-112.

63: TAHERI, Shahrad, et al. Short sleep duration is associated with reduced leptin, elevated ghrelin, and increased body mass index. *PLoS medicine*, 2004, 1.3: e62.

64: MÔNICO-NETO, M., et al. Resistance exercise: A non-pharmacological strategy to minimize or reverse sleep deprivation-induced muscle atrophy. *Medical hypotheses*, 2013.

65: POLESEL, Daniel N., et al. Obesity, Dyslipidemia, and Sleep Disorders Obesity, Dyslipidemia, and Sleep Disorders Complexity Requires Complementary Analysis. *CHEST Journal*, 2013, 143.4: 1187-1188.

66: BAIK, Inkyung, et al. Sleep fragmentation affects LDL-cholesterol and adipocytokines independent of food intake in rats. *Sleep and Biological Rhythms*, 2013.

67: HEGSTED, D. Mark. Energy needs and energy utilization. *Nutrition reviews*, 1974, 32.2: 33-38.

68: BODEN, Guenther. Role of fatty acids in the pathogenesis of insulin resistance and NIDDM. *Diabetes*, 1997, 46.1: 3-10.

69: CONSOLAZIO, C. Frank, et al. Metabolic aspects of acute starvation in normal humans (10 days). *The American journal of clinical nutrition*, 1967, 20.7: 672-683.

70: MORAN, Lisa Jane; NORMAN, Robert John. The obese patient with infertility: a practical approach to diagnosis and treatment. *Nutrition in Clinical Care*, 2002, 5.6: 290-297.

71: CHAKRABARTI, Partha, et al. Insulin inhibits lipolysis in adipocytes via the evolutionary conserved mTORC1-Egr1-ATGL-mediated pathway. *Molecular and cellular biology*, 2013.

72: THOMAS, Elizabeth A., et al. Eating-related behaviors and appetite during energy imbalance in obese-prone and obese-resistant individuals. *Appetite*, 2013.

73: DAVIS, Caroline. From Passive Overeating to "Food Addiction": A Spectrum of Compulsion and Severity. *ISRN Obesity*, 2013, 2013.

74: DEURENBERG-YAP, M., et al. The paradox of low body mass index and high body fat percentage among Chinese, Malays and Indians in Singapore. *BODY COMPOSITION AND DIET OF CHINESE, MALAYS AND INDIANS IN SINGAPORE*, 2000, 69.

75: TOMIYAMA, A. Janet, et al. Low calorie dieting increases cortisol. *Psychosomatic medicine*, 2010, 72.4: 357-364.

76: TREMBLAY, A., et al. Adaptive thermogenesis can make a difference in the ability of obese individuals to lose body weight. *International Journal of Obesity*, 2012, 37.6: 759-764.

77: BLUNDELL, John E., et al. Role of resting metabolic rate and energy expenditure in hunger and appetite control: a new formulation. *Disease models & mechanisms*, 2012, 5.5: 608-613.

78: WELLS, J. C. K. Obesity as malnutrition: the dimensions beyond energy balance. *European journal of clinical nutrition*, 2013, 67.5: 507-512.

79: BARTHEL, Andreas; SCHMOLL, Dieter. Novel concepts in insulin regulation of hepatic gluconeogenesis. *American Journal of Physiology-Endocrinology And Metabolism*, 2003, 285.4: E685-E692.

80: MALINAUSKAS, Brenda M., et al. Dieting practices, weight perceptions, and body composition: a comparison of normal weight, overweight, and obese college females. *Nutr J*, 2006, 5.11.

81: SHEA, J. L., et al. Body fat percentage is associated with cardiometabolic dysregulation in BMI-defined normal weight subjects. *Nutrition, Metabolism and Cardiovascular Diseases*, 2012, 22.9: 741-747.

82: SHAH, Nirav R.; BRAVERMAN, Eric R. Measuring adiposity in patients: the utility of body mass index (BMI), percent body fat, and leptin. *PloS one*, 2012, 7.4: e33308.

83: SCHWARTZ, Michael W.; SEELEY, Randy J. Neuroendocrine responses to starvation and weight loss. *New England Journal of Medicine*, 1997, 336.25: 1802-1811.

84: ATA, Rheanna N.; THOMPSON, J. Kevin. Weight bias in the media: A review of recent research. *Obesity Facts*, 2010, 3.1: 41-46.

85: SAMUEL, Varman T.; SHULMAN, Gerald I. Mechanisms for insulin resistance: common threads and missing links. *Cell*, 2012, 148.5: 852-871.

86: OHKAWARA, Kazunori, et al. Effects of increased meal frequency on fat oxidation and perceived hunger. *Obesity*, 2013, 21.2: 336-343.

87: LUKE, A.; SCHOELLER, D. A. Basal metabolic rate, fat-free mass, and body cell mass during energy restriction. *Metabolism*, 1992, 41.4: 450-456.

88: RANZENHOFER, Lisa M., et al. Pre-Meal Affective State and Laboratory Test Meal Intake in Adolescent Girls with Loss of Control Eating. *Appetite*, 2013.

89: KRISTELLER, Jean; WOLEVER, Ruth Q.; SHEETS, Virgil. Mindfulness-Based Eating Awareness Training (MB-EAT) for Binge Eating: A Randomized Clinical Trial. *Mindfulness*, 2013, 1-16.

90: LE STUNFF, Catherine; BOUGNÈRES, Pierre. Early changes in postprandial insulin secretion, not in insulin sensitivity, characterize juvenile obesity. *Diabetes*, 1994, 43.5: 696-702.

91: GAILLIOT, Matthew T.; BAUMEISTER, Roy F. The physiology of willpower: Linking blood glucose to self-control. *Personality and Social*

Psychology Review, 2007, 11.4: 303-327.

92: GERICH, JOHN E., et al. Hypoglycemia unawareness. *Endocrine Reviews*, 1991, 12.4: 356-371.

93: HUNT, Linda M.; BROWNER, Carole H.; JORDAN, Brigitte. Hypoglycemia: Portrait of an illness construct in everyday use. *Medical Anthropology Quarterly*, 1990, 4.2: 191-210.

94: KAHN, Barbara B., et al. Obesity and insulin resistance. *Journal of Clinical Investigation*, 2000, 106.4: 473-481.

95: BJÖRNTORP, Per. Fatty acids, hyperinsulinemia, and insulin resistance: which comes first?. *Current opinion in lipidology*, 1994, 5.3: 166-174.

96: BERTHELSON, Per, et al. Acute exercise and starvation induced insulin resistance. In: *Medicine & Science In Sports & Exercise, 2012, S498 Vol. 44 No. 5 Supplement. 2661.* 2012. p. 2661.

97: MARTINS, Amanda R., et al. Mechanisms underlying skeletal muscle insulin resistance induced by fatty acids: importance of the mitochondrial function. *Lipids in Health and Disease*, 2012, 11.1: 1-11.

98: YUZEFOVYCH, Larysa V., et al. Mitochondrial DNA damage and dysfunction, and oxidative stress are associated with endoplasmic reticulum stress, protein degradation and apoptosis in high fat diet-induced insulin resistance mice. *PloS one*, 2013, 8.1: e54059.

99: MARCELINO, Helena, et al. A Role for Adipose Tissue De Novo Lipogenesis in Glucose Homeostasis During Catch-up Growth A Randle Cycle Favoring Fat Storage. *Diabetes*, 2013, 62.2: 362-372.

100: KERSTEN, Sander. Mechanisms of nutritional and hormonal regulation of lipogenesis. *EMBO reports*, 2001, 2.4: 282-286.

101: CHAKRABARTI, Partha, et al. Insulin inhibits lipolysis in adipocytes via the evolutionary conserved mTORC1-Egr1-ATGL-mediated pathway. *Molecular and cellular biology*, 2013.

102: LIZUNOV, Vladimir A., et al. Impaired Tethering and Fusion of

GLUT4 Vesicles in Insulin-resistant Human Adipose Cells. *Diabetes*, 2013.

103: HEILBRONN, L.; SMITH, S. R.; RAVUSSIN, E. Failure of fat cell proliferation, mitochondrial function and fat oxidation results in ectopic fat storage, insulin resistance and type II diabetes mellitus. *International Journal of Obesity*, 2004, 28: S12-S21.

104: GINSBERG, Henry N., et al. Insulin resistance and cardiovascular disease. *Journal of Clinical Investigation*, 2000, 106.4: 453-458.

105: GARG, Abhimanyu; MISRA, Anoop. Hepatic steatosis, insulin resistance, and adipose tissue disorders. *Journal of Clinical Endocrinology & Metabolism*, 2002, 87.7: 3019-3022.

106: SHULMAN, Gerald I., et al. Cellular mechanisms of insulin resistance. *Journal of Clinical Investigation*, 2000, 106.2: 171-176.

107: REAVEN, Gerald M. Role of insulin resistance in human disease. *Diabetes*, 1988, 37.12: 1595-1607.

108: LANGIN, Dominique. Adipose tissue lipolysis as a metabolic pathway to define pharmacological strategies against obesity and the metabolic syndrome. *Pharmacological Research*, 2006, 53.6: 482-491.

109: DELARUE, Jacques; MAGNAN, Christophe. Free fatty acids and insulin resistance. *Current Opinion in Clinical Nutrition & Metabolic Care*, 2007, 10.2: 142-148.

110: GARG, Abhimanyu; MISRA, Anoop. Hepatic steatosis, insulin resistance, and adipose tissue disorders. *Journal of Clinical Endocrinology & Metabolism*, 2002, 87.7: 3019-3022.

111: KELLEY, David E., et al. Skeletal muscle fatty acid metabolism in association with insulin resistance, obesity, and weight loss. *American Journal of Physiology-Endocrinology And Metabolism*, 1999, 277.6: E1130-E1141.

112: BROWN, Guy C. Control of respiration and ATP synthesis in mammalian mitochondria and cells. *Biochem. J*, 1992, 284: 1-13.

113: BREMER, J. The role of carnitine in intracellular metabolism. *Journal of clinical chemistry and clinical biochemistry. Zeitschrift fur klinische Chemie und klinische Biochemie*, 1990, 28.5: 297-301.

114: AL, Rodriguez Amaral Almeida, et al. Carnitine supplementation fails to maximize fat mass loss induced by endurance training in rats. *Annals of nutrition and metabolism*, 2004, 48.2: 90-94.

115: KOVES, Timothy R., et al. Mitochondrial overload and incomplete fatty acid oxidation contribute to skeletal muscle insulin resistance. *Cell metabolism*, 2008, 7.1: 45-56.

116: YU, Chunli, et al. Mechanism by which fatty acids inhibit insulin activation of insulin receptor substrate-1 (IRS-1)-associated phosphatidylinositol 3-kinase activity in muscle. *Journal of Biological Chemistry*, 2002, 277.52: 50230-50236.

117: DASHTY, Monireh. A quick look at biochemistry: carbohydrate metabolism. *Clinical biochemistry*, 2013.

118: MUOIO, Deborah M.; KOVES, Timothy R. Skeletal muscle adaptation to fatty acid depends on coordinated actions of the PPARs and PGC1α: implications for metabolic disease. *Applied Physiology, Nutrition, and Metabolism*, 2007, 32.5: 874-883.

119: NGUYEN, Patrick, et al. Liver lipid metabolism. *Journal of animal physiology and animal nutrition*, 2008, 92.3: 272-283.

120: COTTER, David G.; SCHUGAR, Rebecca C.; CRAWFORD, Peter A. Ketone body metabolism and cardiovascular disease. *American Journal of Physiology-Heart and Circulatory Physiology*, 2013, 304.8: H1060-H1076.

121: TSATSOULIS, Agathocles, et al. Insulin resistance: An adaptive mechanism becomes maladaptive in the current environment—An evolutionary perspective. *Metabolism*, 2012.

122: HAMMARSTEDT, Ann, et al. Adipose tissue dysregulation and reduced insulin sensitivity in non-obese individuals with enlarged abdominal adipose cells. *Diabetol Metab Syndr*, 2012, 4.1: 42.

123: P. M. Catalano, L. Presley, J. Minium, and S. H. D. Mouzon, "Fetuses of obese mothers develop insulin resistance in utero," Diabetes Care, vol. 32, no. 6, pp. 1076–1080, 2009.

124: JOHANNSEN, Darcy L., et al. Metabolic slowing with massive weight loss despite preservation of fat-free mass. *Journal of Clinical Endocrinology & Metabolism*, 2012, 97.7: 2489-2496.

125: HOLLOSZY, John O. Exercise-induced increase in muscle insulin sensitivity. *Journal of Applied Physiology*, 2005, 99.1: 338-343.

126: HEATH, G. W., et al. Effects of exercise and lack of exercise on glucose tolerance and insulin sensitivity. *Journal of Applied Physiology*, 1983, 55.2: 512-517.

127: SNIJDERS, Tim, et al. A single bout of exercise activates skeletal muscle satellite cells during subsequent overnight recovery. *Experimental physiology*, 2012, 97.6: 762-773.

128: WADDEN, Thomas A., et al. Lifestyle Modification for Obesity New Developments in Diet, Physical Activity, and Behavior Therapy. *Circulation*, 2012, 125.9: 1157-1170.

129: WILLIS, Leslie H., et al. Effects of aerobic and/or resistance training on body mass and fat mass in overweight or obese adults. *Journal of Applied Physiology*, 2012, 113.12: 1831-1837.

130: WENGER, Howard A.; BELL, Gordon J. The interactions of intensity, frequency and duration of exercise training in altering cardiorespiratory fitness. *Sports Medicine*, 1986, 3.5: 346-356.

131: TAN, Ben. THERAPEUTIC LIFESTYLE CHANGES: EXERCISE & WEIGHT CONTROL.

132: JEFFERY, Robert W., et al. Physical activity and weight loss: does prescribing higher physical activity goals improve outcome?. *The American journal of clinical nutrition*, 2003, 78.4: 684-689.

133: TOWNSEND, Jeremy R., et al. EXCESS POST-EXERCISE OXYGEN CONSUMPTION (EPOC) FOLLOWING MULTIPLE EFFORT SPRINT AND MODERATE AEROBIC

EXERCISE. *Kineziologija*, 2013, 45.1: 16-21.

134: MAGKOS, Faidon, et al. Relationship between adipose tissue lipolytic activity and skeletal muscle insulin resistance in nondiabetic women. *Journal of Clinical Endocrinology & Metabolism*, 2012, 97.7: E1219-E1223.

135: FOSTER-SCHUBERT, Karen E., et al. Effect of Diet and Exercise, Alone or Combined, on Weight and Body Composition in Overweight-to-Obese Postmenopausal Women. *Obesity*, 2012, 20.8: 1628-1638.

136: MCDONAGH, M. J. N.; DAVIES, C. T. M. Adaptive response of mammalian skeletal muscle to exercise with high loads. *European journal of applied physiology and occupational physiology*, 1984, 52.2: 139-155.

137: GELIEBTER, Allan, et al. Effects of strength or aerobic training on body composition, resting metabolic rate, and peak oxygen consumption in obese dieting subjects. *The American journal of clinical nutrition*, 1997, 66.3: 557-563.

138: DOLEZAL, Brett A.; POTTEIGER, Jeffrey A. Concurrent resistance and endurance training influence basal metabolic rate in nondieting individuals. *Journal of applied physiology*, 1998, 85.2: 695-700.

139: CARLSON, B. M.; FAULKNER, J. A. The regeneration of skeletal muscle fibers following injury: a review. *Medicine and science in sports and exercise*, 1983, 15.3: 187.

140: MERO, A. A., et al. Resistance training induced increase in muscle fiber size in young and older men. *European journal of applied physiology*, 2013, 113.3: 641-650.

141: EBENBICHLER, G. R., et al. Load-dependence of fatigue related changes in tremor around 10 Hz. *Clinical neurophysiology: official journal of the International Federation of Clinical Neurophysiology*, 2000, 111.1: 106.

142: SALTIN, B., et al. Skeletal muscle blood flow in humans and its regulation during exercise. *Acta physiologica scandinavica*, 1998, 162.3: 421-436.

143: CLARKSON, Priscilla M.; NOSAKA, Kazunori; BRAUN, Barry. Muscle function after exercise-induced muscle damage and rapid adaptation. *Medicine and science in sports and exercise*, 1992, 24.5: 512-520.

144: ORMSBEE, Michael J.; ARCIERO, Paul J. Detraining Increases Body Fat and Weight and Decreases V [Combining Dot Above] O2peak and Metabolic Rate. *The Journal of Strength & Conditioning Research*, 2012, 26.8: 2087-2095.

145: HUNTER, Gary R.; MCCARTHY, John P.; BAMMAN, Marcas M. Effects of resistance training on older adults. *Sports medicine*, 2004, 34.5: 329-348.

146: HUNTER, Gary R., et al. Resistance training increases total energy expenditure and free-living physical activity in older adults. *Journal of Applied Physiology*, 2000, 89.3: 977-984.

147: SOPHER, Jodie. WEIGHT-LOSS ADVERTISING TOO GOOD TO BE TRUE: ARE MANUFACTURERS OR THE MEDIA TO BLAME?. *Cardozo Arts & Ent LJ*, 2005, 22: 933-933.

148: BØRSHEIM, Elisabet; BAHR, Roald. Effect of exercise intensity, duration and mode on post-exercise oxygen consumption. *Sports Medicine*, 2003, 33.14: 1037-1060.

149: ROSSATO, L. G., et al. Synephrine: from trace concentrations to massive consumption in weight-loss. *Food and chemical toxicology: an international journal published for the British Industrial Biological Research Association*, 2011, 49.1: 8.

150: WASSE, Lucy K., et al. The effect of ambient temperature during acute aerobic exercise on short term appetite, energy intake and plasma acylated ghrelin in recreationally active males. *Applied Physiology, Nutrition, and Metabolism*, 2013, ja.

151: HALSE, Rhiannon E., et al. Postexercise water immersion increases short-term food intake in trained men. *Med. Sci. Sports Exerc*, 2011, 43.4: 632-638.

152: GROFF, Diane G.; LUNDBERG, Neil R.; ZABRISKIE, Ramon B. Influence of adapted sport on quality of life: Perceptions of athletes with cerebral palsy.*Disability & Rehabilitation*, 2009, 31.4: 318-326.

153: JACKSON, Erica M. STRESS RELIEF: The Role of Exercise in Stress Management. *ACSM's Health & Fitness Journal*, 2013, 17.3: 14-19.

154: MOYLAN, S., et al. Exercising the worry away: how inflammation, oxidative and nitrogen stress mediates the beneficial effect of physical activity on anxiety disorder symptoms and behaviours. *Neuroscience & Biobehavioral Reviews*, 2013.

155: FARRELL, Stephen W.; FINLEY, Carrie E.; GRUNDY, Scott M. Cardiorespiratory fitness, LDL cholesterol, and CHD mortality in men. *Med Sci Sports Exerc*, 2012, 44.11: 2132-7.

156: AHMED, Haitham M., et al. Effects of physical activity on cardiovascular disease. *The American journal of cardiology*, 2012, 109.2: 288-295.

157: INTLEKOFER, K. A.; COTMAN, C. W. Exercise Counteracts Declining Hippocampal Function in Aging and Alzheimer's Disease. *Neurobiology of disease*, 2012.

158: BEATRIZ MOTTA, Alicia. The role of obesity in the development of polycystic ovary syndrome. *Current pharmaceutical design*, 2012, 18.17: 2482-2491.

159: GLINA, Sidney; SHARLIP, Ira D.; HELLSTROM, Wayne JG. Modifying risk factors to prevent and treat erectile dysfunction. *The journal of sexual medicine*, 2013, 10.1: 115-119.

160: DESPRES, J. P., et al. Loss of abdominal fat and metabolic response to exercise training in obese women. *American Journal of Physiology-Endocrinology And Metabolism*, 1991, 261.2: E159-E167.

161: IWAMOTO, J. Effects of Physical Activity on Bone: What type of Physical Activity and how much is Optimal for Bone Health. *J Osteopor Phys Act*, 2013, 1: e101.

162: KIRN, Dylan R.; FIELDING, Roger A. Weight Loss and Physical Activity in Obese Older Adults: Impact on Skeletal Muscle and Bone. In: *Nutritional Influences on Bone Health: 8th International Symposium.*

Springer London, 2013. p. 31-41.

163: YOSHIOKA, M., et al. Impact of high-intensity exercise on energy expenditure, lipid oxidation and body fatness. *International journal of obesity and related metabolic disorders: journal of the International Association for the Study of Obesity*, 2001, 25.3: 332-339.

164: BLAIR, Steven N.; CONNELLY, Jon C. How much physical activity should we do? The case for moderate amounts and intensities of physical activity. *Research quarterly for exercise and sport*, 1996, 67.2: 193-205.

165: HANSEN, Kent; SHRIVER, Tim; SCHOELLER, Dale. The effects of exercise on the storage and oxidation of dietary fat. *Sports Medicine*, 2005, 35.5: 363-373.

166: ROSENKILDE, Mads, et al. Body fat loss and compensatory mechanisms in response to different doses of aerobic exercise—a randomized controlled trial in overweight sedentary males. *American Journal of Physiology-Regulatory, Integrative and Comparative Physiology*, 2012, 303.6: R571-R579.

167: ARAGON, Alan Albert, et al. Nutrient timing revisited: is there a post-exercise anabolic window?. *Journal of the International Society of Sports Nutrition*, 2013, 10.1: 5.

168: FOLKOW, Björn, et al. Blood flow in the calf muscle of man during heavy rhythmic exercise. *Acta physiologica Scandinavica*, 1971, 81.2: 157-163.

169: BANGSBO, Jens; HELLSTEN, Ylva. Muscle blood flow and oxygen uptake in recovery from exercise. *Acta physiologica scandinavica*, 1998, 162.3: 305-312.

170: BØRSHEIM, Elisabet; BAHR, Roald. Effect of exercise intensity, duration and mode on post-exercise oxygen consumption. *Sports Medicine*, 2003, 33.14: 1037-1060.

171: JANKOVIC, Aleksandra, et al. Endocrine and Metabolic Signaling in Retroperitoneal White Adipose Tissue Remodeling during Cold Acclimation.*Journal of obesity*, 2013, 2013.

172: PAN, D. A., et al. Skeletal muscle triglyceride levels are inversely related to insulin action. *Diabetes*, 1997, 46.6: 983-988.

173: CHEUVRONT, Samuel N., et al. Water-deficit equation: systematic analysis and improvement. *The American journal of clinical nutrition*, 2013, 97.1: 79-85.

174: HAMILTON, C. L. Interactions of food intake and temperature regulation in the rat. *Journal of comparative and physiological psychology*, 1963, 56.3: 476.

175: DOUCET, Barbara M.; LAM, Amy; GRIFFIN, Lisa. Neuromuscular electrical stimulation for skeletal muscle function. *The Yale journal of biology and medicine*, 2012, 85.2: 201.

176: MAURIÈGE, P., et al. Weight loss and regain in obese individuals: a link with adipose tissue metabolism indices?. *Journal of physiology and biochemistry*, 2013, 1-9.

177: CARPENTER, Catherine L., et al. Body Fat and Body-Mass Index among a Multiethnic Sample of College-Age Men and Women. *Journal of obesity*, 2013, 2013.

178: FOSTER, Gary D., et al. A randomized trial of a low-carbohydrate diet for obesity. *New England Journal of Medicine*, 2003, 348.21: 2082-2090.

179: ECKEL, Robert H., et al. Understanding the Complexity of Trans Fatty Acid Reduction in the American Diet American Heart Association Trans Fat Conference 2006: Report of the Trans Fat Conference Planning Group. *Circulation*, 2007, 115.16: 2231-2246.

180: MOZAFFARIAN, Dariush, et al. Trans fatty acids and cardiovascular disease.*New England Journal of Medicine*, 2006, 354.15: 1601-1613.

181: DHAKA, Vandana, et al. Trans fats—sources, health risks and alternative approach-A review. *Journal of food science and technology*, 2011, 48.5: 534-541.

182: L'ABBÉ, M. R., et al. Approaches to removing trans fats from the food supply in industrialized and developing countries. *European Journal of Clinical Nutrition*, 2009, 63: S50-S67.

183: CATHARINO, Rodrigo Ramos, et al. Characterization of vegetable oils by electrospray ionization mass spectrometry fingerprinting: classification, quality, adulteration, and aging. *Analytical chemistry*, 2005, 77.22: 7429-7433.

184: SCHLEIFER, David. The perfect solution: How trans fats became the healthy replacement for saturated fats. *Technology and culture*, 2012, 53.1: 94-119.

185: ARONIS, Konstantinos N.; KHAN, Sami M.; MANTZOROS, Christos S. Effects of trans fatty acids on glucose homeostasis: a meta-analysis of randomized, placebo-controlled clinical trials. *The American journal of clinical nutrition*, 2012, 96.5: 1093-1099.

186: MENSINK, Ronald P.; KATAN, Martijn B. Effect of dietary trans fatty acids on high-density and low-density lipoprotein cholesterol levels in healthy subjects. *New England Journal of Medicine*, 1990, 323.7: 439-445.

187: MICHA, R.; MOZAFFARIAN, D. Trans fatty acids: effects on cardiometabolic health and implications for policy. *Prostaglandins, Leukotrienes and Essential Fatty Acids*, 2008, 79.3: 147-152.

188: LOPEZ-GARCIA, Esther, et al. Consumption of trans fatty acids is related to plasma biomarkers of inflammation and endothelial dysfunction. *The Journal of nutrition*, 2005, 135.3: 562-566.

189: KUMMEROW, Fred A. The negative effects of hydrogenated trans fats and what to do about them. *Atherosclerosis*, 2009, 205.2: 458-465.

190: ONG, A. S. H.; GOH, S. H. Palm oil: a healthful and cost-effective dietary component. *Food & Nutrition Bulletin*, 2002, 23.1: 11-22.

191: KEYS, Ancel, et al. The seven countries study: 2,289 deaths in 15 years. *Preventive medicine*, 1984, 13.2: 141-154.

DIANA ARTENE

192: PRIOR, Ian A., et al. Cholesterol, coconuts, and diet on Polynesian atolls: a natural experiment: the Pukapuka and Tokelau island studies. *The American journal of clinical nutrition*, 1981, 34.8: 1552-1561.

193: NESS, A. R.; SMITH, G. Davey; HART, C. Milk, coronary heart disease and mortality. *Journal of epidemiology and community health*, 2001, 55.6: 379-382.

194: CONQUER, Julie A., et al. Effect of supplementation with dietary seal oil on selected cardiovascular risk factors and hemostatic variables in healthy male subjects. *Thrombosis research*, 1999, 96.3: 239-250.

195: FERRIÈRES, Jean. The French paradox: lessons for other countries. *Heart*, 2004, 90.1: 107-111.

196: HAYEK, T., et al. Dietary fat increases high density lipoprotein (HDL) levels both by increasing the transport rates and decreasing the fractional catabolic rates of HDL cholesterol ester and apolipoprotein (Apo) AI. Presentation of a new animal model and mechanistic studies in human Apo AI transgenic and control mice. *Journal of Clinical Investigation*, 1993, 91.4: 1665.

197: ELIASSON, B., et al. LDL-cholesterol versus non-HDL-to-HDL-cholesterol ratio and risk for coronary heart disease in type 2 diabetes. *European journal of preventive cardiology*, 2013.

198: WILLERSON, James T.; RIDKER, Paul M. Inflammation as a cardiovascular risk factor. *Circulation*, 2004, 109.21 suppl 1: II-2-II-10.

199: WELTY, Francine K. How Do Elevated Triglycerides and Low HDL-Cholesterol Affect Inflammation and Atherothrombosis?. *Current cardiology reports*, 2013, 15.9: 1-13.

200: SACKS, Frank M.; KATAN, Martijn. Randomized clinical trials on the effects of dietary fat and carbohydrate on plasma lipoproteins and cardiovascular disease. *The American journal of medicine*, 2002, 113.9: 13-24.

201: Yu S, Derr J, Etherton TD, Kris-Etherton P. Plasma cholesterol-predictive equations demonstrate that stearic acid is neutral and monounsaturated fatty acids are hypocholesterolemic. *Am J Clin Nutr.* 1995; 61:1129-1139.

202: BONANOME, Andrea; GRUNDY, Scott M. Effect of dietary stearic acid on plasma cholesterol and lipoprotein levels. *New England Journal of Medicine*, 1988, 318.19: 1244-1248.

203: DENKE, Margo A.; GRUNDY, Scott M. Effects of fats high in stearic acid on lipid and lipoprotein concentrations in men. *The American journal of clinical nutrition*, 1991, 54.6: 1036-1040.

204: MURSU, Jaakko, et al. Dark chocolate consumption increases HDL cholesterol concentration and chocolate fatty acids may inhibit lipid peroxidation in healthy humans. *Free Radical Biology and Medicine*, 2004, 37.9: 1351-1359.

205: LIEBERMAN, Shari; ENIG, Mary G.; PREUSS, Harry G. A review of monolaurin and lauric acid: natural virucidal and bactericidal agents. *Alternative & Complementary Therapies*, 2006, 12.6: 310-314.

206: AMARASIRI, W. A. D. L. Coconut fats. *Ceylon Medical Journal*, 2006, 51.2: 47-51.

207: HAUG, Anna; HOSTMARK, Arne T.; HARSTAD, Odd M. Bovine milk in human nutrition–a review. *Lipids Health Dis*, 2007, 6.25: 1-16.

208: PEETERS, A., et al. Past and future of European grasslands. The challenge of the CAP towards 2020. In: *Grassland-a European resource? Proceedings of the 24th General Meeting of the European Grassland Federation, Lublin, Poland, 3-7 June 2012*. Polskie Towarzystwo Łakarskie (Polish Grassland Society), 2012. p. 17-32.

209: HU, Frank B. Are refined carbohydrates worse than saturated fat?. *The American journal of clinical nutrition*, 2010, 91.6: 1541-1542.

210: MATHEWS, Edward H.; ESPACH, Johanna; LIEBENBERG, Leon. The effect of smoking on blood glucose and coronary heart disease. *Systems engineering investigation into the effects of different lifestyle factors on chronic diseases*, 2012, 230.

211: ORTH-GOMÉR, Kristina, et al. Stress reduction prolongs life in women with coronary disease the Stockholm Women's Intervention Trial for Coronary Heart Disease (SWITCHD). *Circulation: Cardiovascular Quality and Outcomes*, 2009, 2.1: 25-32.

212: VAN CRAENENBROECK, Emeline M.; CONRAADS, Viviane M. On cars, TVs, and other alibis to globalize sedentarism. *European heart journal*, 2012, 33.4: 425-427.

213: LOGUE, Jennifer, et al. Obesity is associated with fatal coronary heart disease independently of traditional risk factors and deprivation. *Heart*, 2011, 97.7: 564-568.

214: SNEL, M., et al. Ectopic fat and insulin resistance: pathophysiology and effect of diet and lifestyle interventions. *International Journal of Endocrinology*, 2012, 2012.

215: STUNKARD, Albert J., et al. An adoption study of human obesity. *New England Journal of Medicine*, 1986, 314.4: 193-198.

216: CAPEAU, J. Insulin resistance and steatosis in humans. *Diabetes & metabolism*, 2008, 34.6: 649-657.

217: LIU, Simin, et al. A prospective study of dietary glycemic load, carbohydrate intake, and risk of coronary heart disease in US women. *The American journal of clinical nutrition*, 2000, 71.6: 1455-1461.

218: HOLMBERG, Sara; THELIN, Anders. High dairy fat intake related to less central obesity: A male cohort study with 12 years' follow-up. *Scandinavian journal of primary health care*, 2013, 31.2: 89-94.

219: CHAVARRO, J. E., et al. A prospective study of dairy foods intake and anovulatory infertility. *Human Reproduction*, 2007, 22.5: 1340-1347.

220: LANDS, Bill. False profits and silent partners in health care. *Nutrition and Health*, 2009, 20.2: 79-89.

221: ILLINGWORTH, D. Roger; HARRIS, William S.; CONNOR, William E. Inhibition of low density lipoprotein synthesis by dietary omega-3 fatty acids in humans. *Arteriosclerosis, Thrombosis, and Vascular*

Biology, 1984, 4.3: 270-275.

222: HARRIS, William S., et al. Dietary omega-3 fatty acids prevent carbohydrate-induced hypertriglyceridemia. *Metabolism*, 1984, 33.11: 1016-1019.

223: BURILLO, Elena, et al. Omega-3 Fatty Acids and HDL. How Do They Work in the Prevention of Cardiovascular Disease? *Current Vascular Pharmacology*, 2012, 10.4: 432-441.

224: Narendran R, Frankle WG, Mason NS, Muldoon MF, Moghaddam B (2012) Improved Working Memory but No Effect on Striatal Vesicular Monoamine Transporter Type 2 after Omega-3 Polyunsaturated Fatty Acid Supplementation. PLoS ONE 7(10): e46832. doi:10.1371/journal.pone.0046832.

225: FLOCK, Michael Ryan, et al. Immunometabolic role of long-chain omega-3 fatty acids in obesity-induced inflammation. *Diabetes/metabolism research and reviews*, 2013.

226: HITCHON, Carol A.; EL-GABALAWY, Hani S. Oxidation in rheumatoid arthritis. *Arthritis Research and Therapy*, 2004, 6: 265-278.

227: PATTERSON, E., et al. Health implications of high dietary omega-6 polyunsaturated fatty acids. *Journal of nutrition and metabolism*, 2012, 2012.

228: HARRIS, William S., et al. Omega-6 fatty acids and risk for cardiovascular disease a science advisory from the American Heart Association Nutrition Subcommittee of the Council on Nutrition, Physical Activity, and Metabolism; Council on Cardiovascular Nursing; and Council on Epidemiology and Prevention. *Circulation*, 2009, 119.6: 902-907.

229: SIMOPOULOS, Artemis P. The importance of the ratio of omega-6/omega-3 essential fatty acids. *Biomedicine & pharmacotherapy*, 2002, 56.8: 365-379.

230: SIMOPOULOS, A. P. Evolutionary aspects of diet, the omega-6/omega-3 ratio and genetic variation: nutritional implications for chronic diseases. *Biomedicine & Pharmacotherapy*, 2006, 60.9: 502-507.

231: EVANS, Lynda Michele; HARDY, Robert William. Optimizing Dietary Fat to Reduce Breast Cancer Risk: Are we there Yet?. *Open Breast Cancer J*, 2010, 2: 108-122.

232: PATTERSON, E., et al. Health implications of high dietary omega-6 polyunsaturated fatty acids. *Journal of nutrition and metabolism*, 2012, 2012.

233: MUHLHAUSLER, Beverly S.; AILHAUD, Gérard P. Omega-6 polyunsaturated fatty acids and the early origins of obesity. *Current Opinion in Endocrinology, Diabetes and Obesity*, 2013, 20.1: 56-61.

234: SANTORO, Nicola, et al. Oxidized fatty acids: A potential pathogenic link between fatty liver and type 2 diabetes in obese adolescents?. *Antioxidants & redox signaling*, 2013.

235: FREEMAN, Marlene P., et al. Omega-3 fatty acids: evidence basis for treatment and future research in psychiatry. *Journal of Clinical Psychiatry*, 2006, 67.12: 1954-1967.

236: DESCHNER, Eleanor E., et al. The effect of dietary omega-3 fatty acids (fish oil) on azoxymethanol-induced focal areas of dysplasia and colon tumor incidence. *Cancer*, 1990, 66.11: 2350-2356.

237: SIMOPOULOS, Artemis P. The importance of the omega-6/omega-3 fatty acid ratio in cardiovascular disease and other chronic diseases. *Experimental Biology and Medicine*, 2008, 233.6: 674-688.

238: PEET, Malcolm; STOKES, Caroline. Omega-3 fatty acids in the treatment of psychiatric disorders. *Drugs*, 2005, 65.8: 1051-1059.

239: CLARK, Stephen R., et al. Characterization of platelet aminophospholipid externalization reveals fatty acids as molecular determinants that regulate coagulation. *Proceedings of the National Academy of Sciences*, 2013, 110.15: 5875-5880.

240: WIJENDRAN, Vasuki; HAYES, K. C. Dietary n-6 and n-3 fatty acid balance and cardiovascular health. *Annu. Rev. Nutr.*, 2004, 24: 597-615.

241: ŁUKASZEWICZ, Marcin; SZOPA, Jan; KRASOWSKA, Anna.

Susceptibility of lipids from different flax cultivars to peroxidation and its lowering by added antioxidants. *Food chemistry*, 2004, 88.2: 225-231.

242: MELLO, Michelle M.; STUDDERT, David M.; BRENNAN, Troyen A. Obesity—the new frontier of public health law. *New England Journal of Medicine*, 2006, 354.24: 2601-2610.

243: SANCHEZ-MUNIZ, Francisco J.; VIEJO, Jesus M.; MEDINA, Rafaela. Deep-frying of sardines in different culinary fats. Changes in the fatty acid composition of sardines and frying fats. *Journal of agricultural and food chemistry*, 1992, 40.11: 2252-2256.

244: GRANDJEAN, Philippe, et al. Cognitive performance of children prenatally exposed to "safe" levels of methylmercury. *Environmental Research*, 1998, 77.2: 165-172.

245: MARRUGO-NEGRETE, José Luis; RUIZ-GUZMÁN, Javier Alonso; DÍEZ, Sergi. Relationship Between Mercury Levels in Hair and Fish Consumption in a Population Living Near a Hydroelectric Tropical Dam. *Biological trace element research*, 2013, 151.2: 187-194.

246: PARILLO, M., et al. A high-monounsaturated-fat/low-carbohydrate diet improves peripheral insulin sensitivity in non-insulin-dependent diabetic patients. *Metabolism*, 1992, 41.12: 1373-1378.

247: SARMAH, Ajit K.; MEYER, Michael T.; BOXALL, Alistair. A global perspective on the use, sales, exposure pathways, occurrence, fate and effects of veterinary antibiotics (VAs) in the environment. *Chemosphere*, 2006, 65.5: 725-759.

248: GYLFE, Erik. Glucose Control of Glucagon Secretion: There Is More to It Than KATP Channels. *Diabetes*, 2013, 62.5: 1391-1393.

249: AMIR, Shimon. Central glucagon-induced hyperglycemia is mediated by combined activation of the adrenal medulla and sympathetic nerve endings. *Physiology & behavior*, 1986, 37.4: 563-566.

250: UNGER, Roger H., et al. The role of aminogenic glucagon secretion in blood glucose homeostasis. *Journal of Clinical Investigation*, 1969, 48.5: 810.

DIANA ARTENE

251: JOHNSTONE, Alexandra M. Safety and efficacy of high-protein diets for weight loss. *Proceedings of the Nutrition Society*, 2012, 71.2: 339.

252: CHALKIADAKI, Angeliki; GUARENTE, Leonard. High-fat diet triggers inflammation-induced cleavage of SIRT1 in adipose tissue to promote metabolic dysfunction. *Cell metabolism*, 2012, 16.2: 180-188.

253: LARK, D. S.; FISHER-WELLMAN, K. H.; NEUFER, P. D. High-fat load: mechanism (s) of insulin resistance in skeletal muscle. *International Journal of Obesity Supplements*, 2012, 2: S31-S36.

254: DAIKHIN, Yevgeny; YUDKOFF, Marc. Ketone bodies and brain glutamate and GABA metabolism. *Developmental neuroscience*, 1998, 20.4-5: 358-364.

255: PICARD, F.; DESHAIES, Y. Inflammation, ectopic fat and lipid metabolism: view from the chair. *International Journal of Obesity Supplements*, 2012, 2: S29-S30.

256: KANG, Hoon Chul, et al. Early-and late-onset complications of the ketogenic diet for intractable epilepsy. *Epilepsia*, 2004, 45.9: 1116-1123.

257: KOVES, Timothy R., et al. Mitochondrial overload and incomplete fatty acid oxidation contribute to skeletal muscle insulin resistance. *Cell metabolism*, 2008, 7.1: 45-56.

258: LEE, Hong Kyu, et al. Mitochondria-Based Model for Fetal Origin of Adult Disease and Insulin Resistance. *Annals of the New York Academy of Sciences*, 2005, 1042.1: 1-18.

259: DUNAIF, Andrea, et al. Insulin resistance and the polycystic ovary syndrome: mechanism and implications for pathogenesis. *Endocrine reviews*, 1997, 18.6: 774-800.

260: KASTURI, Sanjay S.; TANNIR, Justin; BRANNIGAN, Robert E. The metabolic syndrome and male infertility. *Journal of andrology*, 2008, 29.3: 251-259.

261: BACH, A. Oxaloacetate deficiency in MCT-induced ketogenesis. *Archives Of Physiology And Biochemistry*, 1978, 86.5: 1133-

1142.

262: BLACK, Mary Helen, et al. High-Fat Diet Is Associated with Obesity-Mediated Insulin Resistance and β-Cell Dysfunction in Mexican Americans. *The Journal of nutrition*, 2013, 143.4: 479-485.

263: SANDVEI, Marit, et al. Sprint interval running increases insulin sensitivity in young healthy subjects. *Archives of Physiology and Biochemistry*, 2012, 118.3: 139-147.

264: JOHNSON, R. H., et al. Metabolic fuels during and after severe exercise in athletes and non-athletes. *The Lancet*, 1969, 294.7618: 452-455.

265: KOESLAG, J. H. Post-exercise ketosis and the hormone response. *Medicine and science in sports and exercise*, 1982, 14.5: 327-334.

266: CHARLES, Joseph C.; HEILMAN, Raymond L. Metabolic acidosis. *Hospital Physician*, 2005, 41.3: 37-42.

267: HALADE, Ganesh V., et al. High fat diet-induced animal model of age-associated obesity and osteoporosis. *The Journal of nutritional biochemistry*, 2010, 21.12: 1162-1169.

268: LUDWIG, David S. The glycemic index. *JAMA: The Journal of the american medical association*, 2002, 287.18: 2414-2423.

269: WOLEVER, T. M., et al. The glycemic index: methodology and clinical implications. *The American journal of clinical nutrition*, 1991, 54.5: 846-854.

270: VEGA-LÓPEZ, Sonia, et al. Interindividual variability and intra-individual reproducibility of glycemic index values for commercial white bread. *Diabetes Care*, 2007, 30.6: 1412-1417.

271: TROUT, David L.; BEHALL, Kay M.; OSILESI, Odutola. Prediction of glycemic index for starchy foods. *The American journal of clinical nutrition*, 1993, 58.6: 873-878.

272: BAO, Jiansong, et al. Prediction of postprandial glycemia and insulinemia in lean, young, healthy adults: glycemic load compared with carbohydrate content alone. *The American journal of clinical nutrition*, 2011, 93.5: 984-996.

273: WOLEVER, T. M., et al. The glycemic index. *World review of nutrition and dietetics*, 1990, 62: 120.

274: BORCZAK, Barbara, et al. Glycaemic response to frozen stored wholemeal-flour rolls enriched with fresh sourdough and whey proteins. *Starch -Stärke*, 2013.

275: ALFENAS, Rita CG; MATTES, Richard D. Influence of glycemic index/load on glycemic response, appetite, and food intake in healthy humans. *Diabetes Care*, 2005, 28.9: 2123-2129.

276: DODD, Hayley, et al. Calculating meal glycemic index by using measured and published food values compared with directly measured meal glycemic index. *The American journal of clinical nutrition*, 2011, 94.4: 992-996.

277: Read some basic information on the digestion process here: http://digestive.niddk.nih.gov/ddiseases/pubs/yrdd/

278: HOLMES, R. The intestinal brush border. *Gut*, 1971, 12.8: 668-677.

279: HOEBLER, C., et al. Physical and chemical transformations of cereal food during oral digestion in human subjects. *British Journal of Nutrition*, 1998, 80: 429-436.

280: WONG, Julia MW; JENKINS, David JA. Carbohydrate digestibility and metabolic effects. *The Journal of nutrition*, 2007, 137.11: 2539S-2546S.

281: BEHRNS, K. E.; SARR, M. G. Diagnosis and management of gastric emptying disorders. *Advances in surgery*, 1994, 27: 233.

282: HUNT, J. N. A possible relation between the regulation of gastric emptying and food intake. *American Journal of Physiology-Gastrointestinal and Liver Physiology*, 1980, 239.1: G1-G4.

283: SEIMON, Radhika V., et al. Gastric emptying, mouth-to-cecum transit, and glycemic, insulin, incretin, and energy intake responses to a mixed-nutrient liquid in lean, overweight, and obese males. *American Journal of Physiology-Endocrinology And Metabolism*, 2013, 304.3: E294-E300.

284: HUNT, J. N.; STUBBS, D. F. The volume and energy content of meals as determinants of gastric emptying. *The Journal of physiology*, 1975, 245.1: 209-225.

285: FLOURIÉ, B. The influence of dietary fibre on carbohydrate digestion and absorption. In: *Dietary Fibre—A Component of Food*. Springer London, 1992. p. 181-196.

286: GUNNERUD, U. J.; ÖSTMAN, E. M.; BJÖRCK, I. M. E. Effects of whey proteins on glycaemia and insulinaemia to an oral glucose load in healthy adults; a dose–response study. *European journal of clinical nutrition*, 2013.

287: KELLER, Ulrich. Dietary proteins in obesity and in diabetes. *International Journal for Vitamin and Nutrition Research*, 2011, 81.23: 125-133.

288: MIDDLETON, Kathryn R.; ANTON, Stephen D.; PERRI, Michal G. Long-Term Adherence to Health Behavior Change. *American Journal of Lifestyle Medicine*, 2013.

289: WILLETT, Walter C.; STAMPFER, Meir J. Current evidence on healthy eating. *Annual review of public health*, 2013, 34: 77-95.

290: SMITH, Kristen. Body Image and the Health of America: Where Do We Go From Here?. 2013.

291: YAMADA-GOTO, N.; KATSUURA, G.; NAKAO, K. A Novel Approach to Obesity from Mental Function. *J Obes Wt Loss Ther*, 2013, 3.167: 2.

292: BUBLITZ, Melissa G.; PERACCHIO, Laura A.; BLOCK, Lauren G. Why did I eat that? Perspectives on food decision making and dietary restraint. *Journal of Consumer Psychology*, 2010, 20.3: 239-258.

293: ROSSETTI, Clara, et al. Evidence for a compulsive-like behavior in rats exposed to alternate access to highly preferred palatable food. *Addiction biology*, 2013.

294: WUTZKE, K. D., et al. Metabolic effects of HAY's diet. *Isotopes in environmental and health studies*, 2001, 37.3: 227-237.

295: SCHEMBRI, Adrian J. *Eating Disorders and Obsessive-Compulsive Disorder: An Examination of Overlapping Symptoms, Obsessive Beliefs, and Associated Cognitive Dimensions.* 2010. PhD Thesis. RMIT University.

296: DE LUCA JR, L. A., et al. Water deprivation and the double-depletion hypothesis: common neural mechanisms underlie thirst and salt appetite. *Brazilian journal of medical and biological research*, 2007, 40.5: 707-712.

297: BENTON, David; BENTON, David. Can artificial sweeteners help control body weight and prevent obesity?. *Nutrition research reviews*, 2005, 18.1: 63-76.

298: BROWN, C. M.; DULLOO, A. G.; MONTANI, J. P. Sugary drinks in the pathogenesis of obesity and cardiovascular diseases. *International Journal of Obesity*, 2008, 32: S28-S34.

299: DHINGRA, Ravi, et al. Soft drink consumption and risk of developing cardiometabolic risk factors and the metabolic syndrome in middle-aged adults in the community. *Circulation*, 2007, 116.5: 480-488.

300: RIESENHUBER, A., et al. Diuretic potential of energy drinks. *Amino Acids*, 2006, 31.1: 81-83.

301: MAUGHAN, Ron J. Fluid and electrolyte loss and replacement in exercise*.*Journal of sports sciences*, 1991, 9.S1: 117-142.

302: BASU, Sanjay, et al. Relationship of Soft Drink Consumption to Global Overweight, Obesity, and Diabetes: A Cross-National Analysis of 75 Countries. *American journal of public health*, 2013, 0: e1-e7.

303: CRESCENZO, Raffaella, et al. Increased hepatic de novo lipogenesis and mitochondrial efficiency in a model of obesity induced by diets rich in fructose. *European journal of nutrition*, 2013, 52.2: 537-545.

304: AEBERLI, Isabelle, et al. Fructose intake is a predictor of LDL particle size in overweight schoolchildren. *The American journal of clinical nutrition*, 2007, 86.4: 1174-1178.

305: EVANS, E. Whitney, et al. Development of a pediatric cariogenicity index. *Journal of public health dentistry*, 2013.

306: MILLARD-STAFFORD, Mindy, et al. Thirst and hydration status in everyday life. *Nutrition reviews*, 2012, 70.s2: S147-S151.

307: VAN DAM, Rob M.; PASMAN, Wilrike J.; VERHOEF, Petra. Effects of coffee consumption on fasting blood glucose and insulin concentrations randomized controlled trials in healthy volunteers. *Diabetes Care*, 2004, 27.12: 2990-2992.

308: KEIJZERS, Gerben B., et al. Caffeine can decrease insulin sensitivity in humans. *Diabetes care*, 2002, 25.2: 364-369.

309: BEAUDOIN, Marie-Soleil, et al. Caffeine ingestion impairs insulin sensitivity in a dose-dependent manner in both men and women. *Applied Physiology, Nutrition, and Metabolism*, 2012, 38.2: 140-147.

310: XU, Wang, et al. Make Caffeine Visible: a Fluorescent Caffeine "Traffic Light" Detector. *Scientific reports*, 2013, 3.

311: BERGER, Terry A.; BERGER, Blair K. Rapid, Direct Quantitation of the Preservatives Benzoic and Sorbic Acid (and Salts) Plus Caffeine in Foods and Aqueous Beverages Using Supercritical Fluid Chromatography. *Chromatographia*, 2013, 1-7.

312: LEE, Yu-Mi, et al. Exposure assessment of caffeine in children's snacks in Korea. *Food Science and Biotechnology*, 2013, 22.3: 865-869.

313: SWITHERS, Susan E. Artificial sweeteners produce the counterintuitive effect of inducing metabolic derangements. *Trends in Endocrinology & Metabolism*, 2013.

314: DE SOUZA, Russell J., et al. Effects of 4 weight-loss diets differing in fat, protein, and carbohydrate on fat mass, lean mass, visceral adipose tissue, and hepatic fat: results from the POUNDS LOST trial. *The American journal of clinical nutrition*, 2012, 95.3: 614-625.

315: WANNAMETHEE, S. Goya; SHAPER, A. Gerald. Alcohol, body weight, and weight gain in middle-aged men. *The American journal of clinical nutrition*, 2003, 77.5: 1312-1317.

316: CONIGRAVE, Katherine M., et al. A prospective study of drinking patterns in relation to risk of type 2 diabetes among men. *Diabetes*, 2001, 50.10: 2390-2395.

317: GOSLAWSKI, Melissa, et al. Binge drinking impairs vascular function in young adults. *Journal of the American College of Cardiology*, 2013.

318: STOCKWELL, Tim, et al. Under-reporting of alcohol consumption in household surveys: a comparison of quantity–frequency, graduated–frequency and recent recall. *Addiction*, 2004, 99.8: 1024-1033.

319: VERSTER, J. C., et al. 1595–The effects of mixing alcohol with caffeinated beverages on subjective intoxication. *European Psychiatry*, 2013, 28: 1.

320: BERGER, Douglas, et al. Alcohol questionnaires and HDL: Screening scores as scaled markers of alcohol consumption. *Alcohol*, 2013.

321: VAN TOL, Arie, et al. Changes in postprandial lipoproteins of low and high density caused by moderate alcohol consumption with dinner. *Atherosclerosis*, 1998, 141: S101-S103.

322: KOIVISTO, Veikko A., et al. Alcohol with a meal has no adverse effects on postprandial glucose homeostasis in diabetic patients. *Diabetes Care*, 1993, 16.12: 1612-1614.

323: CALIXTO, J. B. Efficacy, safety, quality control, marketing and regulatory guidelines for herbal medicines (phytotherapeutic agents). *Brazilian Journal of Medical and Biological Research*, 2000, 33.2: 179-189.

324: FIRENZUOLI, Fabio, et al. Current issues and perspectives in herbal hepatotoxicity: a hidden epidemic. *Internal and emergency medicine*, 2013, 1-3.

325: IZZO, Angelo A.; ERNST, Edzard. Interactions between herbal medicines and prescribed drugs. *Drugs*, 2009, 69.13: 1777-1798.

326: ANG-LEE, Michael K.; MOSS, Jonathan; YUAN, Chun-Su. Herbal medicines and perioperative care. *JAMA: the journal of the American Medical Association*, 2001, 286.2: 208-216.

327: WHITING, Peter W.; CLOUSTON, Andrew; KERLIN, Paul. Black cohosh and other herbal remedies associated with acute hepatitis. *Medical Journal of Australia*, 2002, 177.8: 440-443.

328: MOREIRA, Ana Paula Lançanova, et al. Determination of diuretics and laxatives as adulterants in herbal formulations for weight loss. *Food Additives & Contaminants: Part A*, 2013, just-accepted.

329: WADDEN, Thomas A.; STUNKARD, ALBERT J.; BROWNELL, KELLY D. Very low calorie diets: their efficacy, safety, and future. *Annals of internal medicine*, 1983, 99.5: 675-684.

330: SKENDER, Martha L., et al. Comparison of 2-year weight loss trends in behavioral treatments of obesity: diet, exercise, and combination interventions. *Journal of the American Dietetic Association*, 1996, 96.4: 342-346.

331: WADDEN, Thomas A.; VAN ITALLIE, Theodore B.; BLACKBURN, George L. Responsible and irresponsible use of very-low-calorie diets in the treatment of obesity. *JAMA: The Journal of the American Medical Association*, 1990, 263.1: 83-85.

332: SOURS, Harold E., et al. Sudden death associated with very low calorie weight reduction regimens. *The American journal of clinical nutrition*, 1981, 34.4: 453-461.

333: BODEN, Guenther. Free fatty acids (FFA), a link between obesity and insulin resistance. *Front Biosca*, 1998, 3: d169-d175.

334: DAVIES, H. J., et al. Metabolic response to low-and very-low-calorie diets. *The American journal of clinical nutrition*, 1989, 49.5: 745-751.

335: WEYER, Christian, et al. Energy metabolism after 2 y of energy restriction: the biosphere 2 experiment. *The American journal of clinical nutrition*, 2000, 72.4: 946-953.

336: FRICKER, Jacques, et al. Energy-metabolism adaptation in obese adults on a very-low-calorie diet. *The American journal of clinical nutrition*, 1991, 53.4: 826-830.

337: TJØNNA, Arnt Erik, et al. Aerobic Interval Training Versus Continuous Moderate Exercise as a Treatment for the Metabolic Syndrome A Pilot Study. *Circulation*, 2008, 118.4: 346-354.

338: BLUNDELL, John E., et al. Cross talk between physical activity and appetite control: does physical activity stimulate appetite?. *Proceedings of the Nutrition Society*, 2003, 62.03: 651-661.

339: WHYTE, Laura J.; GILL, Jason MR; CATHCART, Andrew J. Effect of 2 weeks of sprint interval training on health-related outcomes in sedentary overweight/obese men. *Metabolism*, 2010, 59.10: 1421-1428.

340: BURGOMASTER, Kirsten A., et al. Similar metabolic adaptations during exercise after low volume sprint interval and traditional endurance training in humans. *The Journal of physiology*, 2008, 586.1: 151-160.

341: PERSEGHIN, Gianluca, et al. Increased glucose transport–phosphorylation and muscle glycogen synthesis after exercise training in insulin-resistant subjects.*New England Journal of Medicine*, 1996, 335.18: 1357-1362.

342: TRAPP, E. G., et al. The effects of high-intensity intermittent exercise training on fat loss and fasting insulin levels of young women. *International journal of obesity*, 2008, 32.4: 684-691.

343: BOUTCHER, Stephen H. High-intensity intermittent exercise and fat loss. *Journal of Obesity*, 2010, 2011.

344: EICHNER, E. Randy. Overtraining: consequences and prevention. *Journal of sports sciences*, 1995, 13.S1: S41-S48.

345: FRADKIN, Andrea J.; GABBE, Belinda J.; CAMERON, Peter A. Does warming up prevent injury in sport?: The evidence from randomised controlled trials?. *Journal of Science and Medicine in Sport*, 2006, 9.3: 214-220.

346: JANZ, Jonathon. Warm-Up, Flexibility, and Cool-Down.

347: UZOGARA, Stella G. The impact of genetic modification of human foods in the 21st century: A review. *Biotechnology Advances*, 2000, 18.3: 179-206.

348: ANAND, S. P.; SATI, N. ARTIFICIAL PRESERVATIVES AND THEIR HARMFUL EFFECTS: LOOKING TOWARD NATURE FOR SAFER ALTERNATIVES.

349: LAWRENCE, Mark. The Food Regulatory System–Is It Protecting Public Health and Safety?. *Food Security, Nutrition and Sustainability*, 2010, 162.

350: PENNISTON, Kristina L.; TANUMIHARDJO, Sherry A. Vitamin A in dietary supplements and fortified foods: Too much of a good thing?. *Journal of the American Dietetic Association*, 2003, 103.9: 1185-1187.

351: SANDSTROM, B., et al. Micronutrient interactions: effects on absorption and bioavailability. *British Journal of Nutrition*, 2001, 85.2: S181.

352: JOHNSTON, Carol S.; HALE, Joanna C. Oxidation of ascorbic acid in stored orange juice is associated with reduced plasma vitamin C concentrations and elevated lipid peroxides. *Journal of the American Dietetic Association*, 2005, 105.1: 106-109.

353: LEE, Seung K.; KADER, Adel A. Preharvest and postharvest factors influencing vitamin C content of horticultural crops. *Postharvest biology and technology*, 2000, 20.3: 207-220.

354: PAPIES, Esther; STROEBE, Wolfgang; AARTS, Henk. Pleasure in the mind: Restrained eating and spontaneous hedonic thoughts about food. *Journal of Experimental Social Psychology*, 2007, 43.5: 810-817.

355: DOWNWARD, Paul; RASCIUTE, Simona. Does sport make you happy? An analysis of the well-being derived from sports participation. *International Review of Applied Economics*, 2011, 25.3: 331-348.

356: HALSTED, Charles H. Dietary supplements and functional foods: 2 sides of a coin?. *The American journal of clinical nutrition*, 2003, 77.4: 1001S-1007S.

357: HODGSON, Jonathan M.; HSU-HAGE, Bridget H.-H.; WAHLQVIST, Mark L. Food variety as a quantitative descriptor of food intake. *Ecology of food and nutrition*, 1994, 32.3-4: 137-148.

358: REDDY, Manju B.; LOVE, Mark. The impact of food processing on the nutritional quality of vitamins and minerals. In: *Impact of processing on food safety*. Springer US, 1999. p. 99-106.

359: RICKMAN, Joy C.; BARRETT, Diane M.; BRUHN, Christine M. Nutritional comparison of fresh, frozen and canned fruits and vegetables. Part 1. Vitamins C and B and phenolic compounds. *Journal of the Science of Food and Agriculture*, 2007, 87.6: 930-944.

360: HOLST, Birgit; WILLIAMSON, Gary. Nutrients and phytochemicals: from bioavailability to bioefficacy beyond antioxidants. *Current opinion in biotechnology*, 2008, 19.2: 73-82.

361: GILLOOLY, M., et al. The effects of organic acids, phytates and polyphenols on the absorption of iron from vegetables. *Br J Nutr*, 1983, 49.3: 331-342.

362: BSC, Sc Noonan. Oxalate content of foods and its effect on humans. *Asia Pacific Journal of Clinical Nutrition*, 1999, 8.1: 64-74.

363: BAKER, David H., et al. Problems and pitfalls in animal experiments designed to establish dietary requirements for essential nutrients. *J. Nutr*, 1986, 116: 2339-2349.

364: VAN DOKKUM, W. Significance of iron bioavailability for iron recommendations. *Biological trace element research*, 1992, 35.1: 1-11.

365: LICHTENSTEIN, Alice H.; RUSSELL, Robert M. Essential nutrients: food or supplements?. *JAMA: the journal of the American Medical Association*, 2005, 294.3: 351-358.

366: HARLAND, BARBARA F. Dietary fibre and mineral bioavailability. *Nutr Res Rev*, 1989, 2: 133-147.

367: ANDERSON, James W.; CHEN, Wen-Julin. Plant fiber. Carbohydrate and lipid metabolism. *The American journal of clinical nutrition*, 1979, 32.2: 346-363.

368: CUMMINGS, John H. Nutritional implications of dietary fiber. *The American journal of clinical nutrition*, 1978, 31.10: S21-S29.

369: HALLBERG, Leif, et al. Calcium: effect of different amounts on nonheme-and heme-iron absorption in humans. *The American journal of clinical nutrition*, 1991, 53.1: 112-119.

370: MOLENDI-COSTE, Olivier; LEGRY, Vanessa; LECLERCQ, Isabelle A. Why and how meet n-3 PUFA Dietary Recommendations?. *Gastroenterology research and practice*, 2010, 2011.

371: HUSSAIN, S. Perwez; HOFSETH, Lorne J.; HARRIS, Curtis C. Radical causes of cancer. *Nature Reviews Cancer*, 2003, 3.4: 276-285.

372: OBERLEY, Larry W. Free radicals and diabetes. *Free Radical Biology and Medicine*, 1988, 5.2: 113-124.

373: KALRA, J.; CHAUDHARY, A. K.; PRASAD, K. Increased production of oxygen free radicals in cigarette smokers. *International journal of experimental pathology*, 1991, 72.1: 1.

374: PIERREFICHE, G.; LABORIT, H. Oxygen free radicals, melatonin, and aging.*Experimental gerontology*, 1995, 30.3: 213-227.

375: PHAM-HUY, Lien Ai; HE, Hua; PHAM-HUY, Chuong. Free radicals, antioxidants in disease and health. *International journal of biomedical science: IJBS*, 2008, 4.2: 89.

376: EL-MOWAFY, Abdalla M. Antioxidant Medications: Facts, Myths and Prospects. *Biochemistry & Analytical Biochemistry*, 2013.

377: Bjelakovic, G., Nikolova, D., Gluud, L. L., Simonetti, R. G., & Gluud, C. (2007). Mortality in randomized trials of antioxidant supplements for primary and secondary prevention. *JAMA: the journal oj the American Medicai Association,297*(8), 842-857.

378: BLOCK, Keith I. Antioxidants and cancer therapy: furthering the debate. *Integrative Cancer Therapies*, 2004, 3.4: 342-348.

379: BOREK, Carmia. Antioxidants and radiation therapy. *The Journai of nutrition*, 2004, 134.11: 3207S-3209S.

380: CHOW, Ching Kuang; CHOW-JOHNSON, Hannah S. Antioxidant Function and Health Implications of Vitamin E. *Open Nutrition Journai*, 2013, 7: 1-6.

381: MILLER, Edgar R., et al. Meta-analysis: high-dosage vitamin E supplementation may increase all-cause mortality. *Annals oj internal medicine*, 2005, 142.1: 37-46.

382: KLEIN, Eric A., et al. Vitamin E and the risk of prostate cancer. *JAMA: the journai oj the American Medicai Association*, 2011, 306.14: 1549-1556.

383: RISTOW, Michael, et al. Antioxidants prevent health-promoting effects of physical exercise in humans. *Proceedings oj the Nationai Academy oj Sciences*, 2009, 106.21: 8665-8670.

384: LIPPMAN, Scott M., et al. Effect of selenium and vitamin E on risk of prostate cancer and other cancers. *JAMA: the journai oj the American Medicai Association*, 2009, 301.1: 39-51.

385: OMENN, Gilbert S., et al. Risk factors for lung cancer and for intervention effects in CARET, the Beta-Carotene and Retinol Efficacy Trial. *Journai oj the Nationai Cancer Institute*, 1996, 88.21: 1550-1559.

386: LIN, Jennifer, et al. Vitamins C and E and beta carotene supplementation and cancer risk: a randomized controlled trial. *Journal oj the Nationai Cancer Institute*, 2009, 101.1: 14-23.

387: BENT, Stephen; KO, Richard. Commonly used herbal medicines in the United States: a review. *The American journai oj medicine*, 2004, 116.7: 478-485.

388: BOLLAND, Mark J., et al. Effect of calcium supplements on risk of myocardial infarction and cardiovascular events: meta-analysis. *BMJ: British Medical Journal*, 2010, 341.

389: GIOVANNUCCI, Edward, et al. A prospective study of calcium intake and incident and fatal prostate cancer. *Cancer Epidemiology Biomarkers & Prevention*, 2006, 15.2: 203-210.

390: DATTA, Mridul; SCHWARTZ, Gary G. Calcium and vitamin D supplementation and loss of bone mineral density in women undergoing breast cancer therapy.*Critical reviews in oncology/hematology*, 2013.

391: HEMILÄ, Harri; CHALKER, Elizabeth. Vitamin C for preventing and treating the common cold. *Cochrane Database Syst Rev*, 2013, 1.

392: MURSU, Jaakko, et al. Dietary supplements and mortality rate in older women: the Iowa Women's Health Study. *Archives of Internal Medicine*, 2011, 171.18: 1625.

393: NAIDU, K. Akhilender. Vitamin C in human health and disease is still a mystery? An overview. *Nutrition Journal*, 2003, 2.1: 7.

394: Directive 2002/46/EC of the European Parliament and of the Council of 10 June 2002 on the approximation of the laws of the Member States relating to food supplements". Eur-lex.europa.eu. Retrieved 2012-12-05.

395: US "Dietary Supplement Health and Education Act of 1994". Fda.gov. 2008-10-15. Retrieved 2012-12-05.

396: JORDAN, Melanie A. Interactions with Drugs and Dietary Supplements Used For Weight Loss. 2013.

397: ABRAHAM, Bincy; SELLIN, Joseph H. Drug-induced diarrhea. *Current gastroenterology reports*, 2007, 9.5: 365-372.

398: IOANNIDES-DEMOS, Lisa L., et al. Safety of drug therapies used for weight loss and treatment of obesity. *Drug safety*, 2006, 29.4: 277-302.

399: Weight Management Market by Services, Supplements, Diet, Equipment and Devices: Global Analysis And Forecast (2007 - 2015) - See more at: http://www.transparencymarketresearch.com/weight-management-market.html#sthash.r8w0YT6T.dpuf

400: FONTANAROSA, Phil B.; RENNIE, Drummond; DEANGELIS, Catherine D. The need for regulation of dietary supplements—lessons from ephedra. *JAMA: the journal of the American Medical Association*, 2003, 289.12: 1568-1570.

401: ALLISON, David B., et al. Alternative treatments for weight loss: a critical review. *Critical reviews in food science and nutrition*, 2001, 41.1: 1-28.

402: FISHER, Jennifer Orlet; BIRCH, Leann L. Eating in the absence of hunger and overweight in girls from 5 to 7 y of age. *The American journal of clinical nutrition*, 2002, 76.1: 226-231.

403: WHITAKER, Robert C., et al. Predicting obesity in young adulthood from childhood and parental obesity. *New England Journal of Medicine*, 1997, 337.13: 869-873.

404: JOHNSON, Susan L.; BIRCH, Leann L. Parents' and children's adiposity and eating style. *Pediatrics*, 1994, 94.5: 653-661.

405: ATTIE, Ilana; BROOKS-GUNN, Jeanne. Development of eating problems in adolescent girls: A longitudinal study. *Developmental Psychology*, 1989, 25.1: 70.

406: GOWERS, Simon G.; SHORE, Alison. Development of weight and shape concerns in the aetiology of eating disorders. *The British Journal of Psychiatry*, 2001, 179.3: 236-242.

407: MCCAFFREY, TRACY A., et al. Dietary determinants of childhood obesity: The role of the family. *children*, 2007, 14: 21.

408: BAUGHCUM, Amy E., et al. Maternal feeding practices and childhood obesity: a focus group study of low-income mothers. *Archives of Pediatrics & Adolescent Medicine*, 1998, 152.10: 1010.

409: ROBINSON, Thomas N., et al. Ethnicity and body

dissatisfaction: Are Hispanic and Asian girls at increased risk for eating disorders?. *Journal of Adolescent Health*, 1996, 19.6: 384-393.

410: VÖGELE, Claus. Etiology of obesity. 2005.

411: FIELD, Alison E., et al. Relation between dieting and weight change among preadolescents and adolescents. *Pediatrics*, 2003, 112.4: 900-906.

412: STROEBE, Wolfgang, et al. Why dieters fail: Testing the goal conflict model of eating. *Journal of Experimental Social Psychology*, 2008, 44.1: 26-36.

413: LARDEUX, Sylvie; KIM, James J.; NICOLA, Saleem M. Intermittent access to sweet high-fat liquid induces increased palatability and motivation to consume in a rat model of binge consumption. *Physiology & behavior*, 2013.

414: RATCLIFFE, Denise; ELLISON, Nell. Obesity and Internalized Weight Stigma: A Formulation Model for an Emerging Psychological Problem. *Behavioural and Cognitive Psychotherapy*, 2013, 1-14.

415: FIELD, Alison E., et al. Peer, parent, and media influences on the development of weight concerns and frequent dieting among preadolescent and adolescent girls and boys. *Pediatrics*, 2001, 107.1: 54-60.

416: BROWNELL, Kelly D., et al. Personal responsibility and obesity: a constructive approach to a controversial issue. *Health Affairs*, 2010, 29.3: 379-387.

417: LUSK, Jayson L.; ELLISON, Brenna. Who is to Blame for the Rise in Obesity?.*Appetite*, 2013.

418: LOEWENSTEIN, George. Confronting reality: pitfalls of calorie posting. *The American journal of clinical nutrition*, 2011, 93.4: 679-680.

419: RODRIGO, Carmen Pérez. Current mapping of obesity. *Nutr Hosp*, 2013, 28.Supl 5: 21-31.

www.ingramcontent.com/pod-product-compliance
Lightning Source LLC
Chambersburg PA
CBHW031501270326
41930CB00006B/201